A Practical G
Quality Interaction with Children
Who Have a Hearing Loss

Editor-in-Chief for Audiology
Brad A. Stach, Ph.D.

A Practical Guide to

Quality Interaction with Children Who Have a Hearing Loss

Morag Clark, M.B.E.

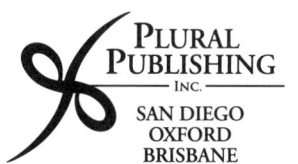

PLURAL
PUBLISHING
INC.
SAN DIEGO
OXFORD
BRISBANE

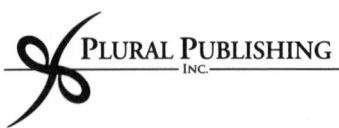

PLURAL PUBLISHING
INC.

5521 Ruffin Road
San Diego, CA 92123

e-mail: info@pluralpublishing.com
Web site: http://www.pluralpublishing.com

49 Bath Street
Abingdon, Oxfordshire OX14 1EA
United Kingdom

ISBN-13: 978-1-59756-112-9
ISBN-10: 1-59756-112-6
Library of Congress Cataloging-in-Publication Data

Clark, Morag.
   A practical guide to quality interaction with children who have a
hearing loss / Morag Clark.
      p. ; cm.
   Includes bibliographical references and index.
   ISBN-13: 978-1-59756-112-9 (softcover)
   ISBN-10: 1-59756-112-6 (softcover)
   1. Hearing disorders in children.   2. Interpersonal relations.
3. Hearing impaired children—Family relationships.   I. Title.
   [DNLM: 1. Hearing Loss.   2. Child.   3. Interpersonal Relations.
4. Language Development.   5. Mainstreaming (Education)
—methods.   6.   Parent-Child Relations.   WV 271 C594p 2006]
RF291.5.C45C553 2006
618.92'09789—dc22

                                            2006021029

Contents

Foreword

The future has never been brighter for infants and young children with hearing loss. After 40 years of tireless, and often thankless, efforts by a small yet committed cadre of professionals with an interest in children with hearing impairment—led by the ageless Marion Downs—we have entered the era of universal newborn hearing screening (UNHS). Technology for automated hearing screening, with otoacoustic emissions (OAEs) and with the auditory brainstem response (ABR), permits quick, accurate, and cost-effective identification of hearing loss in infants within hours after their birth. UNHS programs are now generally supported by official policy in most developed countries, and rapidly expanding throughout the world. In recent years, the application of automated OAE and ABR measurement, in combination, has led to adequate low "refer" rates (<4%) for newborn hearing screening and more rapid identification of infants most likely to have a permanent hearing impairment. Infants who do not pass a hearing screening within days after birth must undergo diagnostic audiologic assessment within months after birth. This important link in the process of early identification and intervention for hearing loss in infants and young children has also been strengthened of late by the application of two techniques for frequency-specific estimation of auditory thresholds: ABRs elicited with tone burst stimulation and the auditory steady state response (ASSR).

Together, tonal activated ABRs and ASSRs provide the essential information on auditory sensitivity necessary for an accurate initial hearing aid fitting for infants, regardless of type or degree of hearing loss, before 6 months. The work of Christie Yoshinago-Itano and colleagues at the University of Colorado has clearly shown that "early" intervention for hearing impairment means within the first 6 months after term birth. That is, a child with hearing impairment—from mild to profound—who benefits from adequate auditory stimulation during the first 6 months after birth is likely to acquire language and speech much as their normal hearing peers. Fortuitously, as the technology for automated hearing screening and accurate diagnosis of hearing loss in infants has evolved rapidly, so has the technology for management. Remarkably small and lightweight digital hearing aids now offer an unprecedented opportunity for precisely amplifying sounds within the speech spectrum. With cochlear implants, the brains of children lacking any response to amplified sound can receive the stimulation necessary for the development of oral language.

A Practical Guide to Quality Interaction with Children Who Have a Hearing Loss is a timely and important contribution to the worldwide effort to provide optimal habilitation for children with auditory dysfunction. In the tradition of Marion Downs, Morag Clark is passionately and totally committed to helping children with hearing impairment develop effective communication abilities with oral language. The peripatetic Ms. Clark has helped to establish educational programs for children with hearing impairment in countries as diverse and distant as Ecuador, Turkey, and South Africa. The odds for success are low. Although the majority of children enrolled in the programs has severe hearing impairment and live in financially impoverished environments, communicative success is not uncommon. In this book, Ms. Clark presents a readable and practical guide to effective education and development of language in children with hearing loss. The overall approach is deceptively simple and logical—encourage early language learning in children with hearing loss as it is stimulated and reinforced in normal hearing children; create a natural and interesting language-learning environment; and put parents and family members in the primary and central role in the process for development of linguistic competence.

A Practical Guide to Quality Interaction with Children Who Have a Hearing Loss is written for all who are involved and invested in the early intervention for children with hearing loss, from parents to professionals. Filled with real-world examples of listening situations and activities, and a lifetime of experience gained in developed and developing countries around the world, this small book fills a large gap in the literature on education and intervention for children with hearing impairment.

James W. Hall, III, Ph.D.
University of Florida
Gainesville, Florida

Acknowledgments

This was a challenging book to write and would not have been possible without the help of several colleagues. I am particularly indebted to Professor Yvonne Csanyi from Budapest and to Sister Anne Tan from Singapore for their help in the analysis of many excerpts of videotape and to Gisela Batliner of Munich for her willingness to comment on the script.

At the same time, I owe a great debt of gratitude to the staff of the Eduplex in Pretoria, South Africa for the freedom I have had to observe and to work with the children with a hearing loss in that program. To Elsie Struwig, Head of Audiology and Parent Guidance, for her patience and readiness to discuss her approach to the work, I am very grateful.

To all the parents and professionals in Turkey, The United Kingdom, South Africa, Singapore, Germany, and Ecuador who have provided photographs to enliven the script I am most grateful.

I thank Dr. James W. Hall, III for his review of the manuscript of this book, and his assistance in bringing it to publication.

Morag Clark, M.B.E.

This book is dedicated to Nico and Anita van der Merve whose vision, turned into reality as a practical program, is changing life for children with a hearing loss in South Africa and beyond.

Introduction

> *"Quality is not something that happens because people are well intentioned."*
> **(van Uden, 1977)**

This book is about *quality* interaction. Professionals who want to implement change in language learning conditions for children with a hearing loss and raise standards of educational programs must realize that, if true quality interaction is to develop, total commitment, careful planning, and effective action are required in addition to good intentions.

This involves:

- the ability to observe and analyze interaction between adults and children
- perseverance when it is difficult to set up the right environment
- awareness of the need for and acceptance of training
- attention to detail in every area of the work.

All of these factors are critical if high standards are to be reached and quality ensured.

Through sharing advice that has proved helpful in many programs throughout the world, this book is a practical guide for professionals seeking to lead children with hearing impairments to fluent, intelligible, spoken language through maximum use of hearing and engaging in quality interaction at the language learning stage.

There are many different approaches to handling the problem of hearing loss in young children and there are as many differences in the young people who eventually leave the various systems after having been handled in very different ways. Advice given in the early years to the parents of children who have a hearing loss has long-lasting effects on the children's development and future lives. Therefore, professionals who first come into contact with families seeking advice on how best to manage a young child who is hearing impaired bear tremendous responsibility for their futures.

Professionals usually offer advice in light of the experience they have had in their particular area of work. The type and degree of experience varies from professional to professional and, in a fast developing field, there can be great differences in the opportunities available for professionals to widen their experience. This is true in many areas of life, but none more so than in work related to the early management of children who are hearing impaired.

Over the course of international work in 12 different countries, it is alarming to discover how many of the young professionals in our field today have had no exposure at all to the possibilities available for children with a hearing loss to achieve when their residual hearing is used to its full potential in an interactive language-learning environment. When children with severe and profound hearing losses are listening well, the quality of their spoken langue often amazes professionals who have not experienced what can happen when active listening skills are fully developed. As expectations are set in the light of our experience, this is a very serious situation.

Developing countries, as opposed to developed countries, may soon lead the way in the future. This is because completely new programs arising in developing countries are not hindered by a heavy weight of tradition from former approaches to the education of children who are deaf (see Appendix A). In Turkey, for example, during the 1980s and 1990s, a strong natural auditory oral (NAO) program was developed—the first of its kind in the entire country. This approach is called "natural" because it seeks to provide the same kind of environment for children with a hearing loss at the language-learning stage, as exists for children with normal hearing. It also emphasizes and uses to the fullest whatever hearing the children may have and is therefore called "auditory." As a result, the children develop spoken language and so it is called "oral."

In Turkey, the program covers the complete range from diagnosis to university entrance for children with severe and profound hearing losses. Very significantly, in addition, a graduate teacher training program of 4 years duration sends out over 30 teachers per year who are thoroughly grounded in the NAO philosophy and its practical application (Clark & Tufekcioglu, 1994). These young teachers never cease to be amazed when visitors, from the United States become excited at the results of the program in Turkey. It is hard for these Turkish teachers to accept that Turkey can lead the way, as they have become so conditioned to importing "expertise" from what they consider to be "developed" countries.

Turkey is no exception. Ecuador is one of the most economically poor countries in the world and yet in Quito, its capital city, there are two vibrant auditory oral programs, one run on private lines and another that works with even the poorest children with a hearing loss. The progress of the children in these programs has given rise to the start of a similar program in Cuenca, a city 10 hours' drive from Quito.

The new South Africa, as a young democracy, is leading the way with one of the most adventurous inclusion programs in the world, in its capital city, Pretoria. The Eduplex, as it is called, has been planned so thoroughly that sufficient support is provided for each learner with a hearing loss and the children are raising the expectations of staff as well as the standards for both children with normal hearing and those with severe and profound hearing losses.

These developments are possible because of major advances in hearing aid technology, audiology, medical science, and psycholinguistics. Before modern hearing aids were available, it was difficult to conceive of the possibility of using the residual hearing of children who had severe or profound hearing losses to lead them to clear, intelligible, spoken language. The speech that children developed in the old oral programs was not always intelligible to strangers and so did not always prepare the young people leaving these programs for life in a hearing world. Modern hearing aids have been widely available in Great Britain since the late 1950s and early 1960s and their quality has improved year by year. When they were first issued, there was tremendous optimism and it was felt that children who were hearing impaired would now learn to listen and to make use of their residual hearing in the language learning process.

For a large number of children, even those with severe and profound hearing losses, this proved to be the case. As they used hearing aids, the children learned to listen and heard the essential characteristics of speech. Backing up these experiences with lip reading, many developed language in the same way as normally hearing children, although in some cases at a slower rate. For an equally large number, however, this was not the case. On analyzing the reasons for these differences, it became clear that the environment in which the hearing aids were used was a major factor in the outcome.

When children with a hearing loss were in an environment that gave them the same linguistic stimulation as children with normal hearing, they were motivated to use their hearing aids and progressed along the road to spoken language, going through the same stages as their normally hearing counterparts. It must be acknowledged that, in spite of appropriate amplification, some children with hearing impairment are still likely to receive reduced auditory cues. As a result, their progress toward fluent spoken language may be delayed, but it need not be deviant if the interactions the child enjoys are similar to those provided for a child with normal hearing at the language learning stage.

For the past 25 years, the author has been involved in advisory work across 14 countries in 5 continents and is, today, still involved in 12. Interest has come from programs that have asked for help in implementing an NAO approach to the development of spoken language in children who have a hearing loss. These requests came from the exposure of personnel in these programs (mainly through excerpts of videotape; Clark, 1985) to a range of young adults with severe and profound hearing losses who have developed fluent, intelligible, spoken language. These young adults come from a wide range of social class, innate ability, and degree of deafness.

The professionals who have asked for help have come from many different countries. They were influenced by their observations of the linguistic independence of groups of young adults who had severe or profound hearing losses and who had been brought up in the NAO approach. As a result, their expectations for the children with whom they were working were raised and they wanted training in this approach. This training has been given in a variety of ways including seminars, courses, and workshops, but mainly, and most effectively, by on site in-service training of staff in the programs concerned. Regular return visits have allowed necessary monitoring of the programs' progress and provided a tremendous learning experience for the author.

The culture and child-rearing patterns of each country are different, and educational systems also vary from country to country. It has, therefore, been necessary to analyze the essential, basic features of the approach so that it could be applied successfully across international boundaries. In the process of this analysis, certain patterns have evolved that highlight elements which can be built into programs universally. In contrast, other features that should be avoided because they detract from the quality of interaction have been identified.

The natural auditory oral approach is a way of life rather than an educational method. It has been well tried and tested in Great Britain since the early 1960s when the author first helped to develop it. At the same time, similar approaches were developing in other parts of the world due to the availability of modern hearing aids (see Appendix A).

Men and women with severe and profound hearing losses who are now now in their 50s and the many younger children who followed them into these programs are a tribute to its success as they can be found living life to the full in society at large. They have linguistic independence, which has enabled them to reach their academic potential and allows them to have privacy because they do not depend on an interpreter. In addition, they are able to choose where they would like to spend their social lives, because they can hold their own in the hearing world and can learn to sign at a later stage if they want to have contact with the Deaf community.

An organization now called DELTA (Deaf Education Through Listening and Talking, formerly NAG) was founded in Great Britain in 1980. It promotes this approach but refers to it as "The Natural Aural Approach." Its literature (DELTA, 1999) highlights the reliability of the approach when it says that:

> It applies current knowledge from the fields of audiology, acoustic phonetics and first language acquisition and has a proven record of achievement in both quality and fluency of speech and in the academic development of children (with a hearing loss).

Requirements for the implementation of the Natural Auditory Oral approach are:

■ The maximum use of residual hearing from the earliest possible age
■ The earliest possible fitting of appropriate amplification (hearing aids, cochlear implants)
■ An environment in which children are surrounded by nothing but normal natural language
■ A sign-free environment
■ The absolute conviction on the part of parents and professionals concerned with the child that children who have a hearing loss have the same innate capacity to develop fluent spoken language as do children with normal hearing, provided that the children with the hearing loss are given the same opportunity.

The "same opportunity" is sometimes difficult to create because knowledge of the presence of a hearing loss in a child often puts pressure on the significant adults in the child's environment to do something "special" to compensate for the hearing loss. Abnormalities in the interaction between an adult and a child with a hearing loss develop all too easily, as will be seen from examples given throughout this book.

> The Natural Auditory Oral approach is based on the fact that, although a child with a hearing loss definitely has special needs, they are not for something different, like a manual means of communication, but rather are for more normality.

The possibility of diagnosing deafness very early, through the developing universal neonatal hearing screening (UNHS) programs in many countries, makes it a matter of urgency to clarify the type of advice to be given to parents of children whose hearing losses are diagnosed when they are very young. Papousek and Papousek (1992) describe how parents may fail to be effective interactive partners with a child who fails to give them the expected responses in communicative situations. Untreated deafness in a child may well result in such a situation and often inhibits the interaction between parent and child.

The impact on educational services that can be expected from the development of UNHS is outlined by McCracken et al. (2005), who sees one of the major challenges to be the need for an "appropriate developmental monitoring within a family centred approach."

If given the correct advice, parents of a child fitted with hearing devices when a few months old can see for themselves that their child can hear. This has a very positive effect on their interaction with the child and increases the possibility of both the child's responsiveness being more normal and the parents learning how to provide a linguistic environment that really is similar to one that a child with normal hearing would enjoy at the language-learning stage.

In the past, little training specifically in dealing with parents whose children's hearing loss was diagnosed at a very young age was available for professionals. The need for training for those working in this area is seen as a matter of urgency (Proctor, Niemeyer, & Compton, 2005).

Robertson and Flexer (2000) support the author's experience when they say, "With the technology and early intervention available today, a child with a hearing loss CAN have the same opportunity as a typically hearing child to develop spoken language, reading and academic skills." Care needs to be taken in this area, however, because overanxiety to establish communication with a child while waiting for a cochlear implant is leading some professionals to advocate the use of sign language at this stage. This shows a lack of understanding of the way in which parents communicate with children who have normal hearing at the prespeech level. Observation shows that there is a time during which communicative behavior is built up before spoken language develops. Given the correct advice, parents of children with a hearing loss build communication skills with their child in the same way, without the use of sign language. The author has found that children who are exposed to sign language before they have a cochlear implant take longer to make full use of the implant than those who are not. They seem to expect to receive information through their eyes and, therefore, it takes more time to condition them to use their hearing fully after they have received the implant. In addition, their body language, influenced by sign language, often takes a long time to become "normal" (e.g.

to get rid of the overexaggerated facial expressions that so often form part of communication by sign).

Children with a hearing loss whose parents are deaf and use sign language as their means of communication in the home are in a different situation. Sign language is their "mother tongue" and the only language to which the children are exposed at home. They come into NAO programs only because the parents want their children to have the opportunity that they themselves missed, of becoming linguistically independent adults. Almost without exception, their listening skills take longer to develop, with a consequent delay in the acquisition of fluent, intelligible, spoken language. It must be realized, however, that only 3% of all children with a hearing loss have two deaf parents (Lynas, Huntington, & Tucker, 1988) and that not all of these children depend on sign language. The number of children worldwide in this category, therefore, is small.

In this controversial field, it is difficult for the uninitiated to understand why all do not turn to making use of everything available today to lead children who are hearing impaired to linguistic independence. For many years, researchers have known of the superior results of young people brought up in wholly auditory oral environments but they have dismissed these results as attainable only by a select group of children from specially favored backgrounds (Paul & Quigley, 1994). Work in developing countries such as Turkey and Ecuador is showing that, provided good foundations are laid and there is adherence to the basic principles outlined in this book, children who are hearing impaired do achieve acceptable levels of functional spoken language and academic success— regardless of their social background, degree of intelligence, or even degree of hearing loss. Spoken language gives them the best possible career opportunities and choice as to where to spend their social lives.

Poor results from the older traditional oral programs undoubtedly lie behind the doubts of many of today's adult deaf who themselves experienced that system. As a result, they found themselves without sufficient fluency in spoken language to feel at home in hearing society. The Natural Auditory Oral approach practiced today is as different from the old oral system as it is from any program that uses signing and it must never be confused with traditional oralism. What must be recognized is the need for constant monitoring to ensure that children with a hearing loss in so-called Natural Auditory Oral programs really do have the same type of linguistic exposure as their hearing counterparts at the language learning stage. In the chapters that follow, ways of attending to detail, the areas to which attention must be directed in the early years, and features that should be avoided are dealt with in detail.

CHAPTER 1

Hearing as the Basis of Development of Spoken Language

> *"The earlier and more efficiently we can allow a child access to meaningful sound with subsequent direction of the child's attention to sound, the better opportunity that child will have to develop spoken language, reading and academic skills."*
>
> **(Robertson & Flexer, 2000, p. 7)**

Due to advances in audiological equipment and techniques, as well as in medical science, it is now a realistic aim to enable almost all children with a hearing loss to develop spoken language primarily through listening rather than through watching. This is best achieved if, at the early stages, parents understand the meaning of the phrase "subsequent direction of the child's attention to sound."

The introduction of universal neonatal hearing screening tests (UNHS) for babies in their first week of life is making it possible for children with a hearing loss to use hearing at a much earlier age than ever before. Follow-up of the babies who fail these screening tests should enable children with a hearing loss to be fitted with appropriate hearing aids by three to six months of age. Such early access to sound means that they are able to develop listening skills at the same time as babies with normal hearing do. It is important that they should because listening is the basis of the development of spoken language. In her Colorado studies, Yoshinago-Itano (2001) found that children born in a hospital with a screening program for hearing loss were 2.6 times more likely to have language within the normal range than those born in a hospital without a screening program.

Early identification of a hearing loss allows early fitting of appropriate hearing aids and early entry into a parent guidance program. The possible future for children with a hearing loss has never been as bright as it is today, but much has to be done if possibilities are to become realities.

Observation of opportunities for the development of listening skills in young children with a hearing loss in the many countries in which the author has worked, for the most part, presents a depressing picture in developed and developing countries alike. Although there are many centers of excellence that can act as models, these centers serve only a minority of the children who need them.

There is a genuine need for a worldwide drive to improve the basic audiological management of young children with a hearing loss. Strauss (2006) suggests that the small number of young children seen each year by individual audiologists probably accounts, at least in part, for the lack of suitable equipment and skill in this area. She suggests that setting up of *centers of excellence*, which could serve as a guide to quality interaction, could be "an effective way to contain costs and yet afford infants the highest quality in early hearing intervention."

The areas that urgently need to be improved are:

- Age of diagnosis of deafness
- Quality of ongoing audiological assessments
- Fitting of two appropriate hearing aids
- Quality and fit of earmolds
- Referral for cochlear implantation where appropriate
- Efficient systems of maintenance of hearing aids and cochlear implants
- Training of parents and professionals in the creation of a listening environment

■ Training of parents and professionals in the development of listening skills that lead to the learning of language

This is not a textbook on audiology. This book addresses only two of the needs listed above: the training of professionals and parents to ensure that maximum use is made of a child's residual hearing by the creation of a good listening environment and the development of listening skills that lead to the development of language.

Training of Professionals

All those working with young children with a hearing loss in a Natural Auditory Oral approach have the duty to ensure that parents of children with a hearing loss are enabled to share responsibility for the development of spoken language of their child. With this goal in mind, one of the initial needs of parents is to become confident in the development of their child's listening skills. It is important for professionals to realize that listening skills are not separate from general learning. They are, in fact, our means of learning because as we learn *to* listen it becomes possible to learn *through* listening. This realization should bring with it a real sense of urgency.

To train parents, professionals themselves may need to be trained in what is available today and how it should be presented to parents. In a large number of the programs in which the author has been involved, too few professionals have had up-to-date knowledge in the area of simple audiology. For some, it is a completely new field; for others it has meant developing a completely new outlook with a resultant raising of expectations.

Conviction That Children Who Are Deaf Can Hear

Basic to all motivation to ensure that hearing devices are well managed is the absolute belief that, with them, the child can hear.

Professionals advising parents must themselves have the experience of observing and identifying responses to sound in young children with a hearing loss who have been properly aided in an environment that promotes the use of hearing. Only then will they be effective in their drive to help parents to understand the importance of "daylong" listening for their child. Those of us who for many years have worked from the basis that, "Deaf children are no longer children who *cannot* hear, but children who *can* learn to listen," are inclined to take it for granted that other professionals share this view. Our excitement about the progress of children who really have learned to listen must not blind us to the need to influence colleagues who have not yet seen the evidence for themselves.

Coupled with the conviction that children who are hearing impaired can learn to listen is the necessity to ensure that an efficient hearing aid and cochlear implant maintenance system is in place because it is essential that the hearing devices function efficiently every day so that the children have the opportunity for daylong listening. Whatever the program, there needs to be a daily system for the checking of the condition of the hearing aids (Figure 1–1).

The author has found a real need for this in the programs in which she has been involved. The following are typical situations.

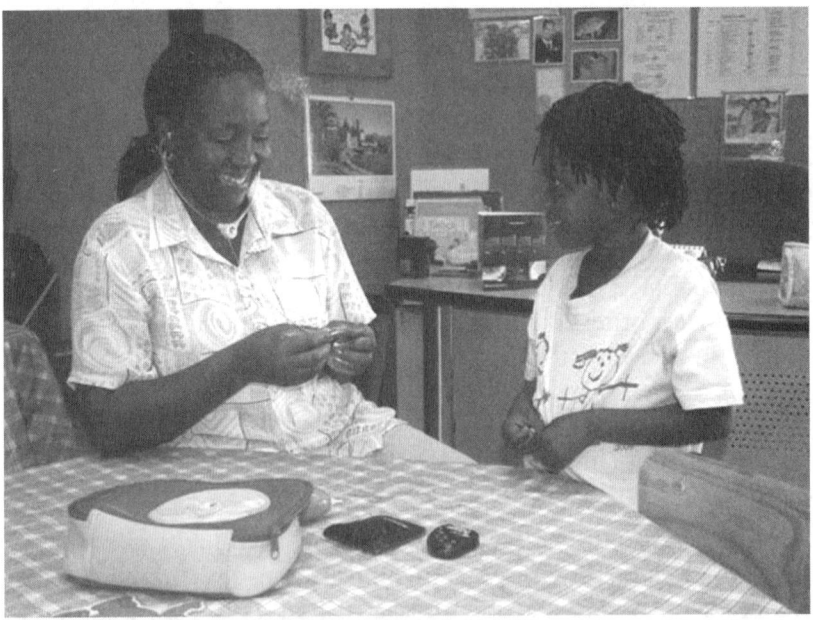

Figure 1–1. *Daily morning checking of hearing aids in South Africa.*

Doctors, Audiologists, and Preschool Professionals

In many countries, parents with children who may have no more than severe hearing losses have been told by some professional that their child is too deaf to benefit from an auditory oral program. Only recently, the mother of a 5-year-old boy, (born with a 105-dB mean hearing loss in the better ear), who is now speaking both German and English fluently, explained how excited she is that this little boy has proved the professionals wrong. She said that, on the day on which the initial diagnosis was made, she was told by the audiologist and doctor that she must understand that the little boy was too deaf to learn to listen, far less speak, and that she must learn to sign immediately. Fortunately, she searched the Internet and found an alternative.

The first professionals to whom parents are introduced when deafness is diagnosed carry a tremendous responsibility because they can have a profound effect on the way in which parents then view their child. In some programs in every country, it has been disturbing to find low expectations in relation to the use of hearing prevalent among those who are the first to advise parents after deafness has been diagnosed. When professionals become convinced that today's situation offers completely new opportunities for the use of hearing, many seek help and come to adopt the Natural Auditory Oral approach. The author has been encouraged by a really dramatic change coming about in several programs, once those running the programs have experienced today's possibilities for listening.

Changing to a Natural Auditory Oral Approach

Changing from Total Communication

The staff of one school using a Total Communication approach, and using it competently, were worried about the poor quality of the spoken language of the pupils. They made tremendous effort and changed completely to a Natural Auditory Oral program with a population of children with severe and profound hearing losses. The change was made gradually over a period of years, beginning with a baby program with children kept separate from the signing children. Today, children in this program are wholly auditory oral in their behavior both in and out of school. They listen extremely well and, with adequate support, many are now included in regular schools. Initially, there was strong resistance to dropping signing by some teachers who were convinced that the children could not hear enough to do without supportive signs. It took several years for the evidence to prove that the children were indeed listening and learning language auditorily, but this change was possible only because the environment in which the children were wearing their hearing aids was completely transformed to meet the requirements of a Natural Auditory Oral approach as outlined in the Introduction.

Changing from Cued Speech

A similar situation occurred in a school using Cued Speech whose students were very "visual" and whose speech was not easily intelligible, because they relied too much on the cues, which are a visual "way in," even though the visual cues are accompanied by spoken language. Some staff in this school actually left the system during the change to a Natural Auditory Oral Approach because they felt that the children would not succeed without the visual cues. In this case, too, the children proved them wrong as they now chatter in fully intelligible, fluent spoken language and have no need of the cues.

Changing from Finger Spelling

Staff in one of the old European Eastern block schools, which used only Finger Spelling without hearing aids, were initially reluctant to believe that use of hearing aids would help their children to develop spoken language. The kindergarten staff volunteered to experiment using hearing aids and a Natural Auditory Oral Approach and the change in the children's communication was so rapid that resistance quickly fell away.

These examples and many other similar cases serve to emphasize the need to ensure that, where there is a will to implement a Natural Auditory Oral Program, the staff dealing with the parents must have a full understanding of and belief in the underlying principles. Before starting any new program or changing the emphasis in an old one, it is necessary to identify staff willing to change and to train them in the new approach.

Guiding Parents

Over 90% of the parents of children with a hearing loss are normally hearing people who have had no experience whatsoever of deafness in a child. Others, who may have had some contact with an adult or young person with a hearing loss, may know nothing of progress that has been made in recent years and the possibilities available today in the handling of a hearing loss in a young child. Others may have been told by a misinformed professional or "Deaf power" advocate that the child belongs to the Deaf world and must learn sign language immediately.

Parents have three main needs in relation to the development of listening skills in their child:

- To realize that their child can hear and learn to listen
- To learn to handle the child's hearing aids or cochlear implant well, to ensure effective binaural hearing wherever possible
- To learn how to create a listening environment

Belief That the Child Can Hear

One of the most positive ways to help parents understand that their child can hear is to demonstrate to them that, with appropriate amplification, their child can hear something. It is not enough merely to tell them the child can hear. They need to observe early auditory responses in the child. Once parents begin to see responses, they are motivated to make sure that the child wears his or her hearing aids during all the waking hours and to be careful about checking the condition of the hearing aids. This often leads to the parents beginning to look more positively on the child.

In many cases, insufficient time is spent on this area in parent guidance programs. Many parents really do need help in recognizing a child's early responses to sound, and they are encouraged when these responses are pointed out to them. It helps to give parents a few pointers to look for at home, for example,

- Did the child stop what he or she was doing when a certain sound was made?
- Did the child look up as if to say, "What was that?"
- Did the child imitate a sound that was made that he did not see?
- Did the child attempt to repeat a word or phrase without eye contact?
- Did the child turn to the sound of a voice, a doorbell, the telephone, or other sound?
- Is the child developing a voice with good pitch, intonation, and rhythm?

One parent, new to an auditory program, was reluctant to admit that there was any change in the behavior of her child when he was wearing his hearing aids. Before she had any faith at all in the hearing aids, it was necessary to point out to her, by means of excerpts of videotape of herself interacting with the child, that when she was chatting with him about a book his eyes were on the pictures and yet he was beginning to imitate the last word of each phrase she used. On another occasion a mother was encouraged when it was pointed out to her that the child stopped playing with his toes when his name was called.

Recently, the mother of a child with problems in addition to deafness came to us with great joy to say, "He really does hear, you know. He now comes when I call him from the kitchen when he is in the next room. I never really believed that would happen with him."

Yet another mother said of her little 18-month-old boy, "I really want everyone to know that my little boy is now part of a world of sound. He listens all the time to everything and wants to talk."

During the parent guidance session, professionals need feedback of this type from parents, who are with the child much more than they are, to learn about the child's responses to sound in the home situation. They then have a much fuller picture of the child's auditory behavior and the fact that they ask the parent about the auditory responses emphasizes the importance that the professional places on the home environment.

Confidence in the Ability to Handle Hearing Devices

Something that has come to light during observation of so many programs in such a variety of countries is that, in many cases, insufficient training is given to parents in the management of whatever amplification devices the child uses. One mother, who had sufficient means to attend a private therapist, transferred to a Natural Auditory Oral program after a year in another program. She had never seen a stetoclip for checking the hearing aids and when offered one to check her child's hearing aids, she put it in the child's ears and asked, "What do I do now?" This was an extreme case, but it takes time for many families to develop the necessary skills and confidence in this area.

For families of limited means, the child's hearing aids may have cost the equivalent of up to 6 months of the family's income, and they are undoubtedly the most valuable things in the home. It is understandable that there should be fear of their being broken. Parents need nonthreatening help and supervision until they are confident that they can check everything adequately and fit the devices onto the child securely. In one country where crime is rampant, parents have to attach the hearing aids in some way to the child's clothing to avoid their being snatched out of the child's ears on a bus or in the street.

Parents should be issued a checking kit at the time that the hearing aids/cochlear implants are issued and should be supervised in its use until they feel confident in their ability to check the hearing devices by themselves. This applies to all families, regardless of economic status. If a child has both a hearing aid and a cochlear implant, it is important for parents to realize the need to check the cochlear implant as regularly as they do the hearing aid.

Ensuring Binaural Hearing

It is a matter of concern to find that some professionals are still content with fitting a child with only one hearing aid initially, although research has shown the importance and benefits of binaural hearing for many years (Markides, 1988). Initially, parents often question the need for two hearing aids or the need for a hearing aid as well as a cochlear implant. Time must be taken immediately after diagnosis to ensure that they understand how important it is for the child to develop directional hearing and that this is possible only when both ears have adequate amplification.

In the early stages of cochlear implant programs, there was reluctance to promote the use of a hearing aid in the nonimplanted ear, but now it is a fully acceptable practice. Dillier (2005) makes a strong case for it on the basis of his research when he says, "Hearing instruments should be used whenever possible to complement the use of cochlear implants and to provide improved sound quality and possibly some localisation abilities."

Providing a Listening Environment

Ours is a noisy world and, as adults, we bring years of experience and of language to a situation in which we have to listen. This is not the case with children. It helps to explain to the parents of a child with a hearing loss that children (with or without a hearing loss) do not hear in the same way as adults. They have to learn to listen and so the conditions in which they learn what sounds mean need to be better for them than for adults. They need to learn the source of various sounds and, in time, to make sense of what is said to them.

The main features of a good listening environment are:

■ **Quiet listening conditions**
  In real life it is not always possible to have quiet listening conditions, but parents should be advised to turn off the radio or television when talking with their child and to interact with the child in the quietest possible conditions. Recently, the author observed a lovely activity between a father and his child who has a profound hearing loss and was wearing his hearing aids. Both were working happily together cleaning the car in front of their house. Unfortunately, it was impossible for the child to hear anything the father said because of the traffic noise on the main road on which the house was situated.

■ **Use of an FM system**
  If an FM system had been in use while the car was being washed, the situation would have been better as the child

would have heard the father's voice at the ear with reduced background noise. Not only hearing aid wearers but also children with cochlear implants should be fitted with FM systems whenever possible.

Ross, M, (1986) himself a wearer of hearing aids, says,

FM systems, in all their various permutations, remain the single most effective way of increasing the speech to noise (S/N) ratio, perhaps the most important factor underlying speech perception perform-ance. Crucial as this can be for adults, it is even more important for hearing impaired children who are in the process of developing speech and language.

The problem for some families in the developing world is the cost of FM systems, which makes them unattainable for many. However, where it is possible to provide an FM system, it should certainly be fitted because it greatly widens the possibilities of a child's learning to listen.

■ **Observance of turn taking by adults**
Sometimes a child is in a situation where two adults are enjoying an activity with him but both are speaking at the same time. This is very confusing to a child because, as an inexperienced listener, it is difficult for the child to know to whom he should attend.

In a parent guidance session recently a 3-year-old boy came in with his mother and grandmother. They had brought material to make sandwiches. It was good to observe that, although both adults were thoroughly involved, only one spoke at a time. Evidence that the child was listening came as he was busy looking at the bread he was buttering and replied, without looking up, when asked what he wanted next, "Peanut butter." In addition, he turned in the direction of the grandmother who had asked the question, thus showing signs of the development of localization of sound. This was a new development, which had to be pointed out to mother and grandmother, both of whom had missed it. With this encouraging input, they left feeling even more confident about the little boy. It is so important that professionals recognize such posi-tive elements and share them with the parents.

Awareness of Environmental Sounds

Children with a hearing loss need to be made aware of environmental sounds and their sources. They need to know not only what makes a sound, but also what does not make sound. Parents should be encouraged to ask regularly, "Did you hear that?" "Do you know what made that noise?" and so on.

When parents and professionals build this routine into their interaction and play with children, the children often take the initiative and are proud to show what they heard spontaneously. A parent recently reported that her two-year-old girl, with a profound hearing loss, who was using two hearing aids well, went running to the door when the dog barked outside, saying, "Woof, woof."

It is very normal and necessary for a family to explore the meaningful noises of their specific environment, but it is not necessary to encourage families to buy specific toys for the purpose of training children to respond to sounds that come from these toys. If a child enjoys a specific toy that makes a noise, by all means that sound should be explored, but it is not necessary to attach sounds to toys bought for the purpose of listening exercises. Everyday life is full of meaningful sound.

■ **Use of an interesting voice of the right intensity**

It is disturbing to find how often in parent guidance sessions that no advice is given to parents about the loudness of the voice. Many parents talk too quietly; occasionally others shout. Right from the start this is an area that should be dealt with in a guidance session so that parents are encouraged to use a normal natural voice so that the child receives a good input on a regular basis.

Parents of young children with normal hearing use a wider range of intonation when talking to them than when talking to adults. Linguists tell us they do this unconsciously to attract the child's attention through the use of an interesting voice. It is reassuring to find that, once parents have confidence in talking to their child with a hearing loss, they also use their voice in this way. It is good to praise them as it helps build their confidence.

■ **Enjoyment of music and rhythm**

Children with a hearing loss enjoy all natural age-appropriate forms of musical activity and greatly benefit from involvement in them. Singing, moving to music, and making music with simple instruments all widen a child's listening experience and help develop a sense of rhythm. Tait (1986) recorded very positive results in a program of singing that she developed for deaf kindergarten children. The author has always included music as a major component of programs in which she has been involved and some of the results can be seen on a videotape entitled Sounds All Around (Clark, 1985; Figure 1–2). If these results could be achieved in 1985, our expectations today should be much higher with the availability of modern amplification systems that provide greatly improved listening opportunities for children with a hearing loss.

When professionals and parents combine to provide an environment in which a child's listening skills can develop to the fullest extent possible, the best foundations are laid for development of intelligible spoken language.

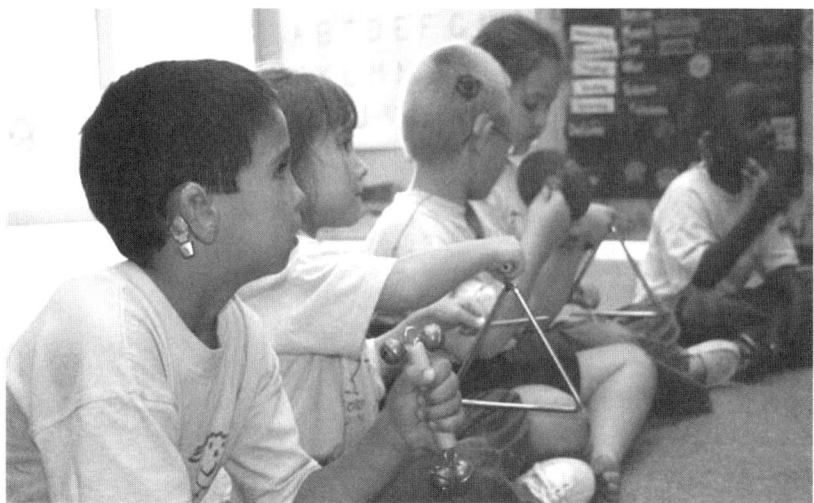

Figure 1–2. *Enjoying playing in the percussion band in South Africa.*

CHAPTER 2

Factors That Detract From the Use of Hearing

Abnormal Visual Cues

In many programs there still exist habits dating from pre-hearing-aid days and these need to be avoided, for example:

- Exaggerated mouth movements of the adult
- Exaggerated facial expressions
- Deliberately drawing attention to the lips—"Watch" instead of "Listen"
- Touching the child instead of calling the name to get attention
- Use of abnormal gestures or sign language
- Exaggerated body language that encourages watching rather than listening.

None of these have any place in a Natural Auditory Oral program.

Possible Pitfalls Related to the Development of Listening Skills

In the course of preparing this book, more than 300 excerpts of videotape were analyzed. They involved parents and professionals seeking to develop spoken language in children with hearing loss as they learned to listen. Many common factors that worked against the development of listening skills were identified. A review of these errors and problems here will help professionals assess both their own skill in this area and those of the parents they advise.

Management of the Child

It must be recognized that, if children's behavior is uncontrolled, they will not use residual hearing to its fullest. Parents, shocked by the knowledge that their child has a hearing loss, often try to compensate by indulging the child. Very often it is necessary to point out to parent guidance program developers that this area must be dealt with before good auditory responses will develop. Until joint attention and cooperative turn-taking have developed, a child will not listen with full attention to input of a conversational partner.

Position

Parents must be made aware that the speaker's distance from the child reduces the signal the child receives from the hearing devices. At the same time, parents are advised that early language develops through the natural interaction of adult and child in the course of daily living. In ordinary homes, this certainly does not take place in a static position, allowing for a constant distance to be kept between speaker and child. An FM system cuts the speaker's distance from the child's ear and solves this problem. It should be used wherever it can be provided.

If, for some reason, a child is auditorily aided only on one side, the speaker should be on the side of the aided ear, wherever possible.

In pre-hearing-aid days parents were advised to make sure the child with hearing loss was watching the parent's face before the parent spoke. There is a tendency for this practice to linger, but this is no longer necessary. Some activities take place naturally when a child is sitting on an adult's knee sharing a book or working side by side in a simple household task. This we see in Figure 2-1 where mother and little girl are chatting as they put washed teacloths back in a drawer. Parents must feel free to adopt a position appropriate for the task when interacting with a child with hearing loss.

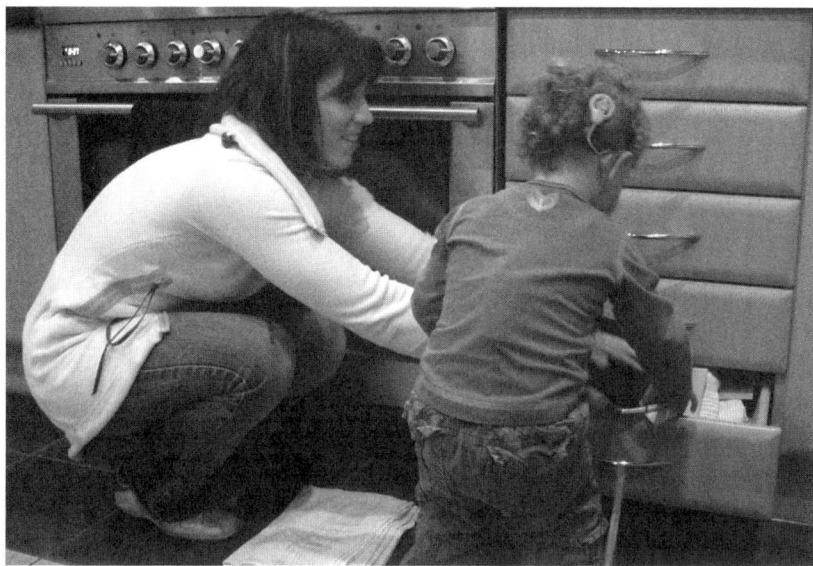

Figure 2–1. *Mother with daughter, age 2 years, 4 months, putting teacloths in a drawer. The child has worn a cochlear implant for 3.5 months.*

Condition of the Hearing Aids or Cochlear Implant

It has been disappointing to find that sessions of Parent Guidance or of individual conversation quite often begin before the hearing devices have been checked (see Figure 2–2). Nonworking or faulty hearing devices certainly inhibit the child's possibility of using hearing to its fullest potential. Several problems interfere with optimal use of amplification:

- Lack of adequate supply and wide enough range of hearing aids or implant processors to allow for the loan of a hearing device of the same model while the child's device is being repaired is a common frustration. An efficient program will always have loaner aids available.
- Poorly fitting ear molds with resultant acoustic feedback are still too common, as are long delays to have them replaced. The author recently spent an afternoon in a program in a developed country where she saw six children, four of whom had "whistling ear molds." It was reported that it would take 2 to 3 weeks to replace them. By contrast, in

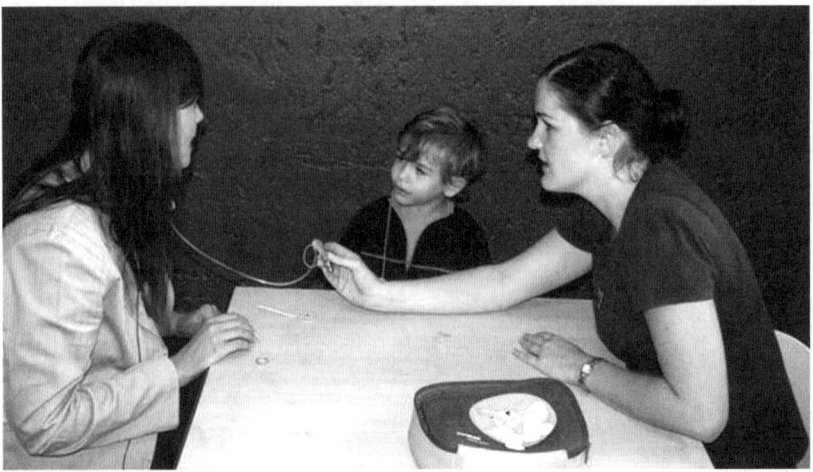

Figure 2–2. *Therapist advising mother on how to check cochlear implants at the start of a Parent Guidance session.*

three developing countries known to the author, there is a 24-hour ear mold replacement service.

- When a child is constantly handling or complaining about an uncomfortably fitting ear mold, lack of investigation can result in the child rejecting the hearing aid. Discomfort should be identified and rectified immediately.

Awareness of Background Noise

- Care must be taken to make sure that no unnecessary background noise is present when an interaction is taking place. During a recent conversation with a therapist, a little boy was tapping his foot against a table. Neither therapist nor child had been aware of this before it was drawn to their attention.
- On another occasion, a therapist's metal bangle was touching the table throughout the whole session and she was quite unaware of it.
- Extraneous background noise of any kind should be avoided. For example, a window should be shut to cut out traffic noise. Ideally windows should be double glazed.

Need to Encourage Child to Listen to Spoken Language

Although it is important for children with hearing loss to experience a wide range of sounds, it must be remembered that we mostly want them to listen to normal spoken language. This knowledge alerts us to certain dangers.

While playing with the young child with hearing loss, it is not sufficient to have toys with buttons producing different sounds that amuse the child. If these are used, there needs to be talk about the kinds of sounds accompanying the activity and anything catching the child's interest. The conversation that takes place around the sounds is then as much a listening activity as the making of the noise.

- Attributing certain sounds to certain toys can limit the development of auditory skills. Quite often sounds made in these situations bear little relation to sounds made by corresponding objects in real life; for example, "Aaah—for Airplane"
- Animal sounds, used by all parents of very young children, are often used excessively in programs designed to enhance listening skills. A parent who recently enrolled her child in an NAO program explained how frustrated she was that for over a year, in the program she had been attending, all "listening exercises" were connected with animal sounds. In a natural program, children do not need "listening exercises" but benefit tremendously from exposure to all normal experiences of sound with which life surrounds them and to which their attention is drawn.
- In daily life, there are so many interesting things to hear that, if parents realize the importance of drawing the child's attention to the various sounds, the children begin to learn through listening.

Avoidance of Overtesting

- Parents are so delighted when their child gives a definite response to a specific sound; for example, there is a tendency for parents to use their child's name continuously as a kind of test. Unless there is a purpose for calling the child, this can lead to the child beginning to ignore the name because nothing happens when he responds. One parent called a child's name five times within 3 minutes and said proudly, "Look, he turns to his name every time."

■ It must be remembered, too, when children with or without hearing loss are absorbed in certain activities, they quite frequently ignore environmental sounds or calls for attention, no matter how often they are repeated. This should be pointed out to avoid parents becoming overly anxious if a child does not respond.

Visual or Tactile Cues

There are two almost opposite situations that cause adults to behave abnormally in relation to additional cues:

■ Prior to fitting the child with a hearing device, the parents have often developed a habit of touching the child to gain attention. This reduces the child's motivation to listen. This is a habit the parents must be assisted in breaking as early as possible.

■ Another similar habit is for adults to wait for eye contact with the child before saying anything. This comes from the mistaken belief that the child must watch as well as listen to hear anything. This habit can slow down the rate at which the child learns to listen and, in addition, breaks the natural flow of interaction.

■ In complete contrast to this is the practice of covering the mouth and denying the child any visual clue. This is far from allowing the child with a hearing loss to have the same opportunity to develop listening skills as the child with normal hearing. We all depend on reading facial expressions when interacting with one another. However, before today's sophisticated hearing devices were available, covering the mouth was introduced as a means of highlighting listening in some programs. This lingers on in many places today. The author has a recent excerpt of videotape showing a child who is listening well with two powerful hearing aids and playing happily on the floor without looking up to respond to questions he answers accurately. During the dialogue his mother, who has transferred from another program in which hand cues were used, covers her mouth with her hand as she says each of the key words. It has become so much of a habit that, even when the child is not looking, she feels the need to deny him the possibility of lip reading, and so her behavior is far from normal.

■ In an NAO approach, parents learn how to avoid giving unnecessary visual cues, while at the same time allowing the child access to all the natural visual cues that would be available to a child with normal hearing. In this approach children with hearing loss independently come to combine listening and looking, as is required in an interactive situation, the same way a child with normal hearing would.

Listening as the Foundation of Intelligible Speech

In pre-hearing-aid days, it was common to include the teaching of speech as a separate subject from the development of language. Lack of ability to access the child's residual hearing, in those days, resulted in the approach to speech as being partly visual and partly tactile.

Advances in hearing aid technology and the availability of cochlear implants have made it possible to have an entirely new perspective in this area. The task can now be thought of as the development of spoken language, rather than the teaching of two separate entities—speech and language—because the "way in" for children with hearing loss can now be predominantly through the ear. Early screening programs that help to identify hearing loss in very young children lead to the early fitting of hearing devices and as a result, children with hearing loss now have the opportunity to develop intelligible spoken language spontaneously at approximately the same time as their normal hearing peers.

Unfortunately, not all children have their hearing loss diagnosed at an early age, and in almost every program, there are children who have come late (after 12–24 months or even much later) to the use of hearing. It often takes longer to lead children in this position to become auditorily aware and to make full use of their residual hearing, but there is no need to return to the old approach. Bearing in mind that the aim is the development of intelligible spoken language, the key to success lies in the input of adults and the number of opportunities the child has to interact with a talking adult.

An interesting study was carried out by Abberton et al. (1987) over a four-year period on children in Birkdale School in England where the approach was wholly Natural Auditory Oral and 87% of the children had hearing losses over 95 dB. It was found that the articulation of the children developed more slowly than, but in the same order as, children with normal hearing.

The temptation for those working with children who have been diagnosed late is to try to "speed things up" by adopting a more formal approach. However, there is a definite need to give these children who come late time to go through the early stages of learning to listen and develop spoken language. There are no shortcuts. The input from the adults in the environment should be that of normal, natural language as well as normal intonation and rhythm. Observation of older children who come late to using their hearing shows that, given the opportunity, many go through the stages of imitation of intonation, rate of utterance, rhythm, and accent before words appear.

In the case of some of these children, however, specific work on the development of auditory skills may be necessary; for example, the following is a program that was outlined by Nevins and Chute (1996). It starts when the child is auditory, with the basic skill being that of mere "detection" of sound, and leads the child as far as possible through the stages of "discrimination" and "identification" to "comprehension."

In their latest book Chute and Nevins (2006), acknowledging the need for systematic attention to be paid to the development of listening skills, still favor the basis for this as their current classroom themes. They suggest "a protocol in which listening is infused into the content themes already a part of the academic demands of the day."

From practical experience, the author has found that this approach serves two purposes:

■ Giving the desired attention to the development of auditory skills
■ Reinforcement of the necessary exposure to the language associated with the theme

In many programs this auditory skill development is built in as part of an individual conversation session for which time is planned daily. Observations provide evidence for the care that must be taken so that excessive anxiety for good results on the part of an adult does not result in long periods of drill. If this happens, tension is apt to creep in, voice quality will suffer, valuable conversational opportunities will be missed.

Even with late beginners we must think of the process as a daylong listening experience, not simply auditory training. As long ago as 1985 Pollack (1985) said, "Sessions of acoustic exercises are not the answer to the child's need. Listening must be a continuous activity."

It is important to be aware that formal speech teaching is still part of many programs. Quite recently one seven-year-old girl, taken out of a group for "individual conversation," was observed practicing the sound "n" in isolation and then in a string of unknown words for a period of 10 minutes. In the end she left with a feeling of failure as the therapist remarked, "I hope you will do that better tomorrow."

This exercise was a holdover from pre-hearing-aid days' practice and is one that must be guarded against in any program seeking to operate on NAO lines today. Even with children who come to hearing late, the focus must always be on something meaningful, in which the child sees some purpose. In addition, the child should leave each individual session with a feeling of success.

The Atmosphere—Expecting to Understand and to Be Understood

The atmosphere in which an interaction takes place is very important. Children are communicative when they feel comfortable with the adult they are interacting with. If there is anxiety and formality on the part of the adult, the child often becomes tense. The atmosphere should be one in which both participants expect to understand each other and be understood so that they are relaxed during the interaction. The child then uses listening to its fullest potential in order to facilitate the sharing of meaning and the understanding of contribution of the conversational partner.

CHAPTER 3

Laying the Foundations of Language Through Daily Living

Children who are hearing impaired now have access to sound. Combine that with their innate capacity to learn spoken language and they are able to go through the same main language learning stages as children with normal hearing. The challenge for those working with children who have a hearing loss is to be convinced of this as they study the environments in which children with normal hearing develop language and then to provide the same opportunities for the children with whom they work.

In most homes, the same things happen at the same time of day on weekdays, Monday to Friday. The routines change on weekends, but the repetitive nature of the day-to-day routines provides real opportunities for consolidation of experiences and the language that accompanies them. Figure 3–1 illustrates just one of the many routine household tasks in which mother and child can share meaning. So much is happening linguistically when parents involve children in the routines of daily living.

It is commonly recognized that parents are the first educators and it is in the home that the child with normal hearing develops fluency in the mother tongue. For any child born with a hearing

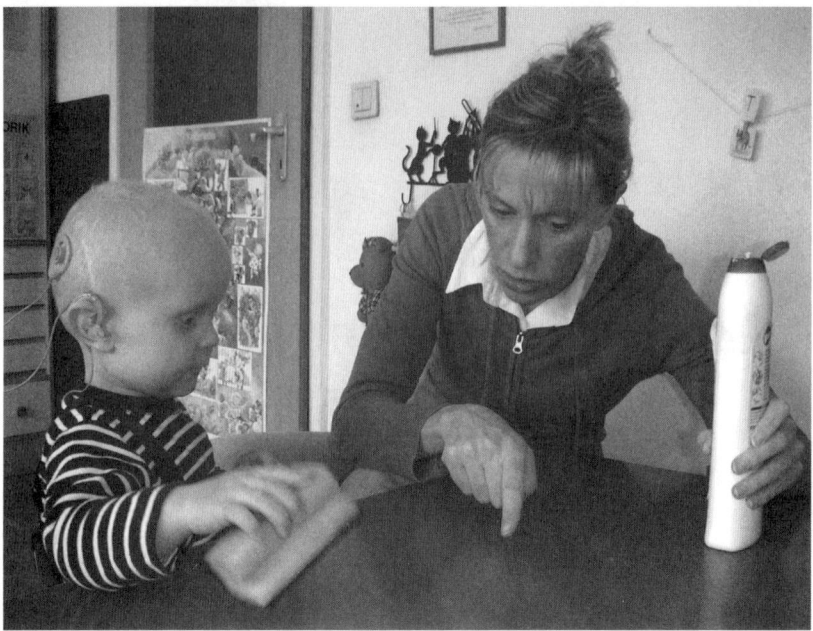

Figure 3–1. *Mother and 18-month-old son (awaiting a second cochlear implant), interacting in an everyday household activity in Germany.*

loss to two normally hearing parents, the mother tongue is the language of the home, namely, spoken language. The daily routine of the home can provide the same opportunity for children with a hearing loss as for those with normal hearing if simple routine situations are developed into language-learning opportunities.

Children with normal hearing develop communicative behavior before they begin to talk. It is important that everyone involved with young children with a hearing loss realizes these children, too, will follow this pattern in their linguistic development. Anxiety about the possible effect of hearing loss sometimes causes those working with young, hearing-impaired children to try to rush ahead with teaching vocabulary before the children have had time to develop communicative behavior. Cole (1992), aware of how dangerous this is, quotes Sugarman (1983) as saying:

> Some preverbal experiences and acquisitions may nonetheless be critical to some aspects of language development. For example, it

may be that, unless children have learned something about communication prior to speaking, they would have little motivation to look for a language to learn.

Cole goes on to identify three fundamental features of discourse that are learned preverbally:

■ Joint reference
■ Turn-taking
■ Signaling of intention.

Joint Reference (Joint Attention)

If there is to be fluent communication, it is necessary for the communicative partners to attend to the same thing. Before a child talks, this sharing often takes place through eye contact and gesture. Parents of children with normal hearing often regulate this by following the child's gaze and chatting about what interests the child. Later, the child comes to follow the parent's gaze. If given the same opportunity, children with a hearing loss follow the same pattern, although for some it may take longer.

The home is full of opportunities for development of joint attention; for example, a mother was dusting a table in the sitting room and chatting to her 18-month-old little girl who had a profound hearing loss. The dialogue went as follows:

Mother, pointing to the side of a bookcase, "Oh, look how dusty this bookcase is."

Child looks where mother points.

Mother looking around, "I need a duster."

Child follows mother's gaze.

Mother, "Oh, here's a nice clean duster"

Child holds out hand for duster, "a—a— a"

Mother handing a second duster to the child, "Oh, you want one too, do you?"

Both mother and child begin to dust the table.

Mother pointing,"You dust that bit and I'll dust here."

Child points to another dusty part of the bookcase.

Mother recognizes this as a nonverbal turn in the communication and says," That's right, it's dusty there too."

The child nods and so the interaction goes on.

In this situation, mother and child were involved in a joint activity and the language used by the mother illustrates that she was following the child's interest in this mundane activity. They were sharing meaning at a very basic level as the little girl was communicating with her mother in a wholly natural, preverbal way. The importance of the linguistic input connected with everyday household chores cannot be overemphasized.

Turn Taking

Repetition of routine interactive experiences in the home is a means of helping to establish turn-taking. Many early parent-child routines are unique and look just like and are fun, but Bruner (1983) maintains that these lay the foundations of later conversation. One mother was found putting small balls down a rubber hose and the child was catching them as they came out the end of the hose. Next the child put a ball down the hose and mother caught it. Not only was this establishing turn-taking, but it was providing repetition of the same language in a meaningful situation: "Pop it in" and "Out it comes" were used throughout, time and time again.

Signaling of Intention

The whole aim of interaction between two people is to convey an idea or meaning from one to the other. Very early on, the baby may not behave with intent, but mothers treat the child's behavior as though it had intent and gradually the child (around 8–10 months) begins to expect certain adult behavior to follow certain behaviors of his or her own.

One mother, looking into the mouth of a four-month-old baby said, "Oh I think I see a little tooth appearing." Immediately the baby gurgled and mother, treating this as agreement said, "Oh, you think so too, do you?"

A one-year-old baby, whose hearing aids had been fitted since she was four months old, pointed to a cupboard and vocalized each time she passed. The mother, taking the pointing with vocalization as a message said, "Oh yes, the chocolate is in there, but it's not for now."

Brown (2002) supports this view when she says, "Even before a child begins to produce recognizable words, there are qualities of interaction between parent and child that are important to assess."

Many people who work with young children with a hearing loss pay lip service to this idea but, in fact, few are relaxed enough to give children time to go through this stage at their own pace. Some children pass through it quite rapidly after receiving their hearing aids, whereas others may take a very long time. When this is really put into practice, it can mean a long period of input during which the child appears to give little response. It is at this time that professionals, who are working with the parents, need the skill to identify very small steps of progress that the child is making and to point these out as progress to the parents. It is very seldom that tiny steps of progress cannot be identified between sessions of Parent Guidance over a period of 6 or 8 weeks if professionals or parents are aware of what to look for.

Two excerpts from the parent guidance of a child who developed slowly, probably on account of late diagnosis, serve to illustrate this point. The child has an average hearing loss in the better ear of 95 dB but did not have this loss diagnosed until 1 year, 9 months. (The value of keeping a longitudinal videotape record of a child's developing language is also illustrated by the mother's comments.)

Excerpt 1—Child Age 2 Years, 1 Month

This was the family's third session of parent guidance.

Report

"Has accepted the hearing aids well—mother reports daylong use.

Mother checks the hearing aids in a capable way.

Mother very disappointed that she could not observe progress when the child was wearing the hearing aids.

No response to sound of any kind observed throughout the session, no eye contact with mother, no vocalizations, difficult to engage in any activity."

Excerpt 2—Same Child Age 2 Years, 4 Months

Three months later—10th session in the program.

Report

"Hearing aids have been very well maintained and child wears them during all his waking hours.

Occasionally turns to his name when called, by hearing alone, but not yet consistently.

Mother is developing interactive play with him—used big beads to string on a lace—child looked up and held out a hand to signify to mother that he wanted the next bead.

- this ensures the development of eye contact
- it is also laying the foundations of turn-taking
- child is beginning to take some initiative in the interaction—on a few occasions directed mother's behavior by pointing
- very quiet, occasional vocalizations heard when child wants another bead."

Mother was depressed because the child was not yet talking. She was shown a videotape of the child from the two sessions recorded above, which illustrated the changes in and development of communicative behavior. She was encouraged and went away feeling much more positive about the child.

The importance of this encouragement cannot be overemphasized. As she left, the mother said, "Without your showing me that, I would have kept on thinking that there was no progress, because

I'm always waiting for him to talk. After seeing these two bits of video, I can see how he has developed in so many ways. Thank you very much." Not all mothers can or will express such feelings, but many do feel disheartened in the early stages after the fitting of the hearing aids and this is an area in which support is urgently needed from the professional.

Busy mothers, especially those in families with no domestic help, often feel guilty that they cannot fit in time every day to sit with the child at a table and "teach the child language." All mothers need to be reassured that their task is not that of "teaching language," but rather that of using the home environment in such a natural way that the child has the opportunity to "learn" language.

It is obvious to many professionals who have had wide experience in the Natural Auditory Oral approach that every situation in the child's life can be a language learning opportunity. The Turkish mother and her child who has a cochlear implant are seen in Figure 3–2 communicating over putting earth in a plant pot. Time and again, the importance of involving the child in household activities

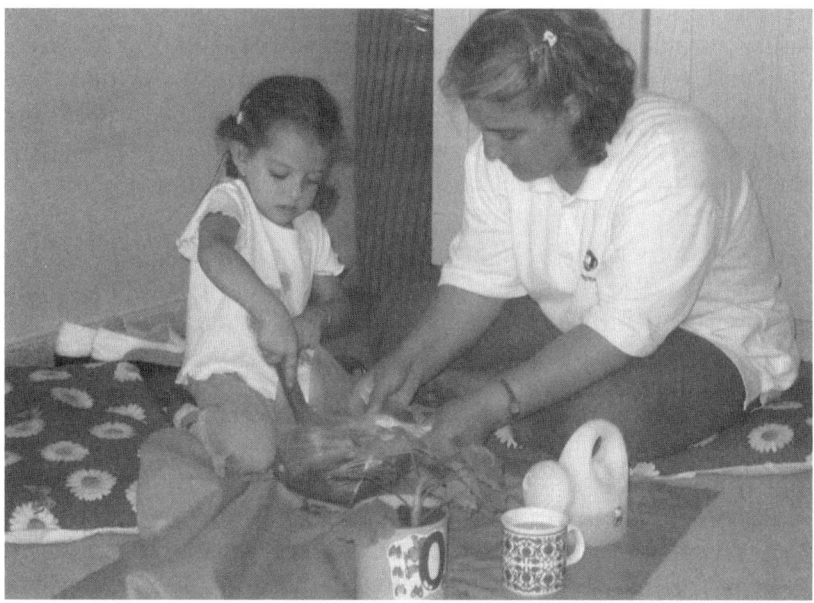

Figure 3–2. A Turkish mother and her little girl with a cochlear implant busily engaged in putting earth in a plant pot.

must be stressed to parents until they begin to take every opportunity the home offers to talk about the daily routine.

At an even more basic level there is the often repeated, very routine situation of changing a diaper. Parents can be encouraged to talk to the child each time and so provide repetitive language, naturally, in a meaningful situation.

The kitchen provides a wealth of opportunities in which to engage children and surround them with meaningful context-related language. General household cleaning tasks often motivate the child to want to take part and thus provide wonderful language-learning opportunities.

We must, however, be careful about the way in which we advise parents to use these occasions. It is also necessary to observe how parents are using them. Two contrasting situations show what parents did after being asked to make soup during the next home visit of the professional. These show how important it is to follow up advice given.

Both families were from the same socioeconomic background and the children had very similar hearing losses. (95 dB to 100 dB loss in the better ear). Both children had their hearing loss diagnosed between 15 and 16 months. Their chronologic ages were within two months of each other (2 years and 2 years, 2 months). The type of early intervention programs in which they had been placed, however, operated in very different ways. As a result, the way in which each child's hearing loss was handled differed. It is important to take the time to analyze two such different situations and to identify what kind of language experience the child is being given. It is then possible to decide whether, in fact, the child is having the basic requirement of "the same opportunity as a child with normal hearing at the language learning stage."

The First Child: Age 2 Years, 2 Months, Fitted with Hearing Aids at 15 Months

Early intervention background: Mother transferred to an NAO program when the child was 2 years old and was finding it difficult to shed the formality of the oral program from which she had come.

Situation: The home kitchen. Child wearing hearing aids and mother using FM system.

Mother was asked to make soup on the professional's visit.

Dialogue:

Mother: "Sit at the table now." (Mother aside to professional—"I make sure he sits at the table every day when I teach him.")

Mother, holding up an onion: "Look, this is an onion. It's an onion. Listen, an onion. What is it?"

Child: No response.

Mother: "Listen again—an onion. Say that for me, an onion"

Child: "u."

Mother: "Onion. Well let's see if we do better with the carrot."

Child holds out his hand for the carrot.

Mother, withdrawing the carrot: "No, listen, this is a carrot, a carrot. Listen, a carrot. What is it?"

Child holds out hand again and says: "a."

Mother: "No, you can't have that yet. We have more here—look" She holds up a leek. "This is a leek. Listen, it's a leek, a leek. What is it?"

Child tries to get off the chair.

Mother: "No you don't. Say leek. Listen, leek!"

Child screams and hits mother.

Mother to professional: "Do you see now that you can't do activity things with him, like you say. He needs the words first and it is so difficult for him to hear and to remember the words, but he is intelligent, I know."

In this situation both mother and child feel like failures.

The questions we have to ask here are:

- Was there any real communication between mother and child?
- Did they enjoy interacting together?
- Was meaning shared?

The answer to all three is a resounding *NO*.

In addition, both mother and child were unhappy and the relationship between them was strained. Mother was disappointed in the child and the child would feel a sense of failure. It is quite clear that this is not the kind of situation in which a normally hearing child learns language and so this child is not having the same opportunity as a hearing counterpart to develop language in a natural way, although the mother is conscientiously setting aside time daily to "teach him language."

The Second Child: Age 2 Years, 0 Months, Fitted with Hearing Aids at 16 Months

Situation: In the home kitchen with the child wearing hearing aids and mother using FM system.

Mother had been in an NAO program since the child was diagnosed.

Dialogue:

Mother, holding a full plastic bag out to the child: "Oh, this bag is heavy, let's see what's inside."

Child runs to look and puts her hand into the bag.

Mother: "That's right, pull one out."

Child pulls out a carrot, points to the dirt on the carrot and pulls a face.

Mother touches the dirt and says: "Oh yes, that carrot's very dirty." Pointing to the sink she goes on "We'll have to wash that carrot."

Child takes it to the draining board of the sink, leaves the carrot there and runs back to mother.

Mother, looking into the bag: "What else have we here?"

Child runs and pulls out some parsley. She smells it. Mother says, "Do you like that smell? That's parsley."

Mother smells it and says: "Mm, I like the smell of parsley too. Look, we can pull the little bits of parsley apart. We'll put all the parsley in this little bowl. You pull some parsley and I'll pull some parsley."

Lots of laughter follows as they pull all the sections of parsley apart.

Mother smells her hands and child copies.

Mother: "Now our hands smell of parsley"

Child, smelling her hands says: "Pa-ly."

Mother: "Yes, that's right. They smell of parsley."

That activity of soup making went on in this way for almost an hour. Vegetables were washed, scraped, and chopped. The child did not once lose interest. What solid foundations for language were being laid in this everyday task! Let's analyze these.

An overview of the whole situation shows clearly that mother and child are really engaged in a joint activity and are sharing meaning in a most natural way. There is absolutely no tension or sense of failure. Each expects to and does understand the other. As yet the little girl has very little actual vocabulary in which to express her ideas, but communication skills have been developed to quite a high level. A more detailed analysis of the interaction shows how this has been achieved. Let's look at this.

1. **Nonverbal behavior**
   The mother's wholly normal, nonverbal behavior helps the child to understand what is meant and expected of her. For example, the mother:

   - holds out the bag toward the child when inviting her to see what is inside
   - puts her hand on the same piece of dirt that the child indicated and so gives the child positive feedback that she has been understood
   - points naturally to the sink to indicate where the carrot will be washed
   - looks into the bag as an indication that they were ready for something else
   - smells the parsley before commenting on it
   - actually pulls a section of parsley apart as she invites the child to follow

- enjoys just laughing with the child
- gives a further experience of the smell by smelling her hands and so the child copies this.

2. **Spoken language input**

A general comment must be that the tone of voice was friendly and encouraging throughout. The spoken language was fluent with all the natural intonation, rhythm, and stress patterns that would be used with a child of similar age who had normal hearing. A more detailed analysis shows:

- A respect for the child in that the mother issues an invitation to join her with,
  "Let's see what's inside"
- Encouragement for the child as her participation is acknowledged,
  "That's right, pull one out"
- An awareness of exactly what the child wanted to convey and the extension of the child's nonverbal utterance by offering the appropriate spoken language.
  "Oh yes. That carrot's very dirty"
- Extension of the idea as well as reinforcement of the word "carrot" as she says,
  "We'll have to wash that carrot."
- Ability to sustain the activity with a simple,
  "What else have we here?"
- The following of the child's interest in the smell of the parsley and the use of the appropriate language connected with this,
  "Do you like that smell? That's parsley. Mm, I like the smell of parsley too."
- The development of the activity so as to reinforce the area in which the child has shown particular interest.
  "Look, we can pull little bits of parsley apart. We'll put all the parsley in this little bowl. You pull some parsley and I'll pull some parsley."
- Further reinforcement with,
  "Now our hands smell of parsley."
- Positive feedback to the child's attempt of, "Pa—ly,"
  "That's right. They smell of parsley."

In the case of these two parents, the responsibility for the difference in the quality of interaction between parent and child lay mainly on the shoulders of the professionals who guided them. After six months in a Natural Auditory Oral program the first mother was able to adapt to a natural approach and built up a warm relationship with her child. The child began to enjoy time with his mother and to develop communication skills before he began to talk. The examination of these two cases calls for serious consideration to be given to the form of Parent Guidance offered to the family of a child with a hearing loss.

CHAPTER 4

Parent Guidance

> *"It can't be said enough—early intervention is critical."*
>
> **(Robertson & Flexer, 2000)**

Hearing loss in young children has long been recognized as a challenge for parents to face alone. In an attempt to address this, early intervention programs have been established in many places around the world, but at the beginning of the 21st century, one cannot claim that there is equal access to these programs for all who need them. In some developing countries, there is little or no help for families who have a child with hearing loss. There is an urgent, worldwide need to establish programs that guide parents who have child with impaired hearing.

The work of Morrison, Rimm-Kauffman, and Pianta (2003) further emphasizes the importance of enhancing parental communication skills. They point out how the quality of mother-child interaction can affect a child's social and academic success.

In many of today's early intervention programs, it is obvious that tradition has created a situation in which professionals working with families of young, hearing-impaired children have come to be looked upon as "the experts," and parents have become dependent on them. This "professional-centered-approach" has led parents to believe that their child will talk if only they, the parents, can model their behavior on that of the professional. It is almost incredible but, as the author travels around the world she finds parents trying to copy the very words used by the professional, for example, "up, up, up—down; whee—; round and round and round, and oh, oh" said with the identical intonation of the professional. This is most unnatural. Every family is unique and parents have their individual styles, which must be retained, unless they are in some way detrimental to the development of spoken language.

It may be helpful to return to the old term of "parent guidance," which has largely been replaced by the term "early intervention" in recent years. "Parent guidance" conjures up a clearer picture of both parent and professional roles. Immediately after diagnosis, parents need entry into a program that will guide them so they are able to manage their hearing-impaired child independently with confidence and competence. Parents must make choices all along the way and the professional should be able to give them enough information of the right kind to ensure that they can make an informed choice.

As the author observes parent guidance programs in many different cultures, she notices that the most effective work is done when professionals manage to establish a relationship with parents that is a partnership.. This is a partnership in which parents are comfortable and can be themselves, not a copy of a therapist.

The Need for a New Focus in Early Intervention Programs

With the UNHS programs developing and identifying children at a very early age, there is a real urgency to train all who work with the parents of these very young children specifically in the developmental stages of young children with normal hearing. A natural approach cannot be implemented any other way. We must ensure that the guidance offered to parents of a child diagnosed very early is age appropriate. It should take into account all the medical and technologic advances of recent years as well as the individual circumstances of each family.

The opportunities available for children diagnosed in the first few weeks or months of life are exciting because early diagnosis allows the family to get help at the optimum age for language learning. There need not be such a delay in language as before.

Therapists used to working with children 2 or 3 years old find themselves in a completely different situation when faced with very young children. They are often at a loss as to how to support the family. Once again it is a matter of following how the parent of a child with normal hearing interacts with the baby in the early months and developing the same simple routines that allow for as normal repetition as possible.

In many programs, there are families whose first language is not that of the community or the language in which the child will be educated. In this situation, it is important to encourage the parents to talk with the hearing-impaired child in the language of the home. A normal language-learning environment can only be created when using a language in which the adult feels comfortable and has flexibility. The emotional bond that builds up between parent and child cannot be established naturally when a parent is hesitant and lacks the expressions used in the mother tongue. The author has a wide range of experience with children with severe and profound hearing losses who have been spoken to in the language of their home only and have later come into educational programs that use a different language. Although their progress initially may be slower in both languages, these children become truly bilingual in school, speaking both the home language and that of the school. For example, in Singapore where there are four different home languages, the program operates in English. A similar situation exists in South Africa where the program caters to both English and Afrikaans, but many of the children come from homes in which an African language such as Zulu, Sotho, or Xhosa is used. There are, in fact, 11 official languages in South Africa.

The early intervention programs that exist worldwide vary tremendously in approach. If we genuinely want children with hearing loss to learn language in the same way as a child with normal hearing, we must examine critically the type of early intervention available to the parents. A young child spends almost all waking hours with the parents or a caregiver, and the parents and caregivers must develop the skill to interact with the child to build language learning opportunities into the daily home routine. Even where the family has access to an early intervention program, the amount of time spent with a professional is minimal. As more and more very young children are diagnosed, there is a real need to reassess early intervention programs. This may often call for a change of focus in that whole area.

In many programs parents are required to observe the therapist at work with the child and often come to believe they must copy the therapist's behavior. This happens because the therapist is seen as the "specialist." Observation of programs around the world shows that professionals often do not act in a way that will really empower parents. This problem seems to arise because of the concept many professionals have about their role in a parent guidance session. Many come into a session with general preset goals, rather than with the desire to focus on *observing the parents and then deciding the needs* of a specific parent-child relationship at a specific language learning stage.

From the start, parents must understand that the professional's task is to observe and to offer advice on the type of interaction that the professional sees them enjoy with the child. Initially, some parents are resistant to this approach because they want the child to receive "therapy" from the professional. They prefer to be observers rather than interact with their own child.

Underlying Principles for Professionals

Every Family Is Unique

The first principle to realize is that every family is unique. It is a privilege to have access to a parent and a very young child. The presence of hearing loss in that child should not mean the family has to alter what would have been its natural child-rearing approach to fit the professional's concept of child rearing. The only time a professional should alter the way a child is managed, is when there is behavior that is inhibiting the development of listening and of spoken language.

Listeners, Not Lecturers

Because of their experience, there are many things that professionals feel parents need to know. There is a temptation to overload families of newly diagnosed children with too much information.

Professionals working in this area must train themselves to be good listeners so they can deal with the immediate concerns of the family. They can then gradually introduce what they feel is important for the family to know.

Some parents find it difficult to voice their concerns and professionals must learn to pick up any information that may be included in chance remarks. Our very questions must be guarded. Positive enquires should be made to parents. They should not be asked outright what worries they have about their child because it suggests we expect them to be worried. A better approach is to ask, "And how has he or she been since we saw you last?" This provides an opportunity for parents to voice both satisfactions and worries and often provides the professional with the opportunity to emphasize the positive at a time when parents may have negative feelings about the child.

Confine the Task to Parent Guidance

The area of parent guidance is broad and professional efforts in this work should be confined to that alone. Professionals who work with children with hearing loss are neither marriage guidance counselors nor social workers; and yet time and again, well-intentioned professionals dabble in areas in which they are not trained. When criticism is voiced, the justification is often that the parents are so wrapped up in their troubles that they can listen to nothing else until they are cleared up. The professional in parent guidance work is responsible for knowing trained people to whom parents can be referred for help with problems other than the child's hearing loss. At the same time, it needs to be recognized that the sooner parents begin interacting with the child, the sooner their confidence grows and communication skills develop.

It is difficult for professionals who have worked in a program dominated by the professional to change. They need to be willing to step back, become observers, and trust parents. They also have problems realizing that parents mostly require mere encouragement to act normally with their child. Some professionals feel very threatened by a natural approach and feel their specialty disappears. They are uncomfortable due to uncertainty about what should replace it. Those who do make the shift usually never want to go back to the more formal way. We now consider how many ways the role of professional may need to change as the Natural Auditory Oral approach has developed.

Suggested Form of a 1-Hour Parent Guidance Session Based on an Observational Model

This is merely a guide and need not be adhered to strictly, but it has been appreciated by young professionals coming into this work as well as by others switching to the observational approach. The timing cannot be adhered to strictly because the needs of both parent and child vary from day to day. The suggested time is a guide to ensure that all parts of a session are covered.

1. (5-10 minutes)—Professional observes parent checking hearing aids or implant and asks how child has been since last visit.
2. (10-15 minutes)—Observes parent interacting with the child.
3. (10-15 minutes)—Professional discusses the observed interaction (this can be included after step 4 or 5, if appropriate).
4. (Approximately 10 minutes)—Professional works with the child.
5. (5-10 minutes)—Professional and parent engage in a joint listening activity often involving music.
6. (Approximately 10 minutes)—Discussion about possible activities between this and the next session of parent guidance. In addition there are always opportunities to discuss how language can be expanded as parent and child engage in interaction related to the daily routine.
7. Writing a report of the session after parent leaves.

Let's look at each of these sections in detail.

Checking the Hearing Device

It is very important for parents to accept full responsibility for efficient functioning of the child's hearing devices. At the start of each session, this quick check highlights its importance and allows the professional to make sure this important task is done routinely.

The author has her own approach to this. To save time, she asks the parent to check one hearing device while she checks the other. A note is made of which ear's device the author checked and on the next visit she asks for the other one, thus ensuring she has listened regularly to both devices. A similar pattern is followed for children with a cochlear implant and a hearing aid in the other ear.

Observing the Parent's Interaction

Parents are asked to bring something from home to use during their time of interaction. The reason for this request is that the professional learns the type of activity in which parent and child engage in the home situation. Some come without anything so it is necessary to have something ready for that situation.

It is very important to ensure that whatever is given to the parent is also available in the home. Recently, the author was in a developing country and the parent was given an elaborate plastic toy. She was very young and she herself had never had access to such a toy as a child. She spent her interaction time almost playing with the toy on her own!

Simple tasks like cleaning shoes, washing socks, making a sandwich or fruit juice, sorting clothes to be washed, or tidying out a cupboard, and so forth, can be replicated in the home. Once parents understand how language can be expanded during such simple activities in the daily home routine, they become active partners in the creation of language-learning opportunities. The Ecuadorian mother seen in Figure 4–1 is involved in the simple preparation of food, which gives her opportunity to use everyday language in context with her child.

If given the wrong advice, parents could turn into teachers who sit the child down to "teach language." This must be avoided.

Pinker (1994) reminds us, in relation to children with normal hearing, that, "Language is a complex, specialized skill that develops in the child spontaneously" and that "language is not something that (parents) teach their children."

If the situation in which the guidance takes place allows, it is good for the professional to observe and listen from outside the room, either by a closed-circuit TV system or through a two-way

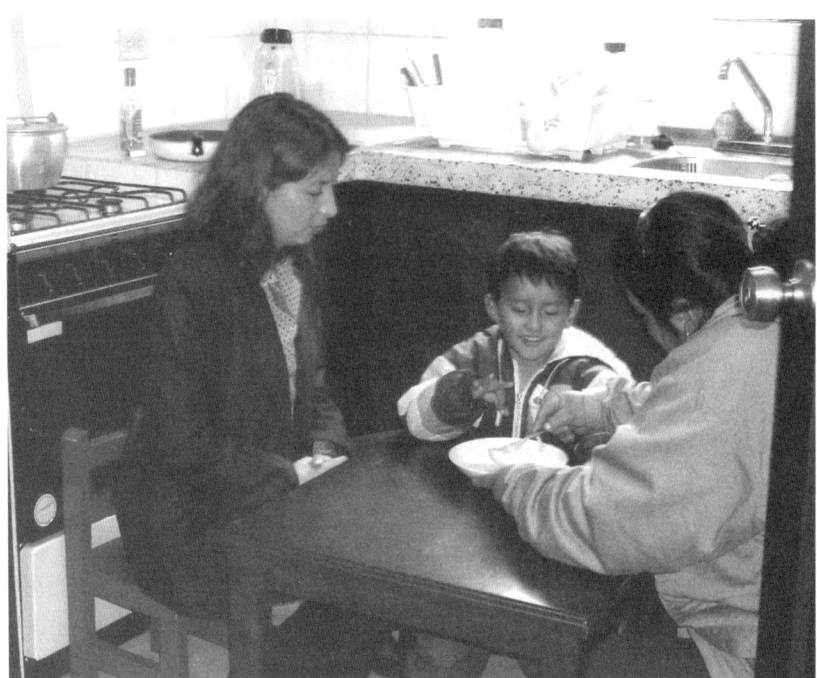

Figure 4–1. *Ecuadorian therapist looks on as a mother and her 4-year-old boy with a severe hearing loss enjoy making scrambled eggs.*

screen. Children do behave differently in situations where another adult is present along with the parent and parents are often self-conscious in the presence of the professional. The most natural setting is that in which parent and child play in a room on their own.

To understand the parents' home situation, it is helpful if some of the guidance can be given in the home. There, the professional can weigh how the parents are placed in relation to extraneous noise, interruptions, and so forth. In many cases, the author has found it necessary to ask for the radio or television to be switched off before the session began as some parents began playing with the child regardless of the background noise. In other cases, neighbors would visit, have a chat, and sit down to watch. In such conditions it is difficult for the child to concentrate on interacting with the parent and the quality of communication is poor. Figure 4–2 shows a therapist observing a common task in the child's home.

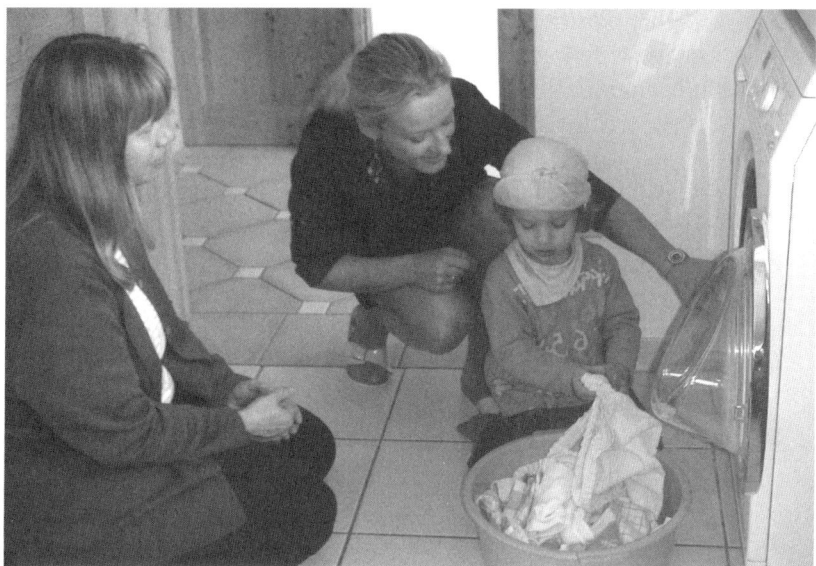

Figure 4–2. *German mother interacting with her two-and-a-half-year-old as they fill the dryer. Therapist is observing.*

Discussion of the Observed Interaction

It must always be remembered that the main aim of parent guidance is to lead parents toward confidence, competence, and independence in handling their hearing-impaired child. It is important to avoid having parents become dependent on therapists or to have them become depressed because the therapist seems more capable than they are. At the same time, it is important to monitor the child's progress and to share this with the parent. Holmans (2005) sees such monitoring as the key to maintaining parent's enthusiasm toward interacting with their child.

Every effort must be made by the professional to praise all positive elements in the interaction and to explain why they were positive. In each parent guidance session, only one feature of what has been observed, should be highlighted to point out change that could lead to improvement. Once parents have been shown their strengths, they are in a receptive mood when offered guidance on how to improve, but it is important not to overload them with advice.

If possible, parent guidance sessions should be videotaped and small sections showing progress should be added to an individual, longitudinal videotape record of the child's developing language. This video record serves different purposes. It allows for:

■ A review of a session and observation in more detail than can be seen while the session is in progress
■ Comparison of the present session with earlier sessions to assess what progress has been made
■ The copying of relevant parts to record progress
■ Parents viewing of the tape so that they can see for themselves the strong and weak points of the interaction
■ The encouragement of parents as they look back and can see progress between the earlier and the present level of the child
■ Training of professionals in the natural approach.

Interaction Between Professional and Child

Placing of professional's interaction with the child after the parent-child interaction is deliberate. In the early stages, after the diagnosis of a child's hearing impairment, parents' self-confidence can be undermined and they often feel intimidated by the "expertise" of a professional. It is better, therefore, for the professional to follow rather than precede the parent in interacting with the child. In addition, this provides an opportunity for the professional to demonstrate practically any change that would improve the parent's interaction.

A mother of three children with hearing loss said that, for her, the most useful part of the guidance sessions was watching the professional work with her child. She felt that this reinforced what she did. Seeing the professional use normal, natural language reassured this mother that she was on the right track and did not need to be doing anything different or special. Also, seeing the child and professional not always understand each other made the mother feel more comfortable when there was a breakdown of communication between herself and the child.

It is usually better for the professional to begin a new activity rather than take over one from the parent, but there are times when the child really and justifiably wants to continue with what the parent has begun. Different activities provide different language experiences and parents gain ideas from observing them, as do professionals from observing creative parents.

Listening Activities, Often Involving Music

It is very important to attend to the development of listening skills in a child with hearing loss. Parents can be encouraged to join in activities that promote better listening, but they often need help initially in creating activities that are suitable. It is worth spending time in a parent guidance session to introduce enjoyable, age-appropriate activities parents can continue at home.

The simple dramatization of stories lends itself to children listening for various voices or specific noises associated with the stories. Rhymes, poems, and simple songs become favorites, as do musical games or simple music and movement sessions.

Parents must understand that these specific listening skill activities help to highlight the use of hearing and are enjoyable in themselves. The most solid work is done in the stimulation of listening to everyday life situations. This is when children are exposed to normal, natural language in meaningful situations.

Discussion of Probable Activities Before the Next Session

Toward the end of a parent guidance session, it is wise to discuss areas of language that might be developed at home before the next session. This does not mean that parents should be given specific vocabulary to "work on," but rather that they should be shown how to expand language around events and activities that will be arising in the home; for example, a visit to the supermarket may be planned. It is not possible to always deal in such detail with an everyday occurrence, but the suggested form below often helps new parents to understand how linguistically valuable such a routine can be.

If the next procedure is followed, good exposure to everyday language comes about naturally.

- Before the visit, parent and child look in the kitchen to see what needs to be bought and discuss who will look for particular items

- Pictures of a few of the items are drawn, talked about, and given to the child who has to look for these items in the supermarket
- Mother herself makes a regular shopping list and talks about this with the child.
- On arrival at the supermarket, the child is responsible for finding the items for which pictures have been drawn
- These are put in a separate bag at the checkout
- On arrival home, time is taken to unpack this bag and to talk about each item and where it has to be put in the kitchen
- When other family members come home or grandma visits, the child tells what has been bought and shows where it is.

In this way, regular household activities are used so the child is exposed to the language in a natural setting in many different ways. There is the opportunity not just to experience and understand it, but also to try to use it.

Home is the place where children with normal hearing are incidentally exposed to many mathematical concepts (e.g., time, money, size, weight, capacity, length, etc.). Children with hearing loss do not overhear as much incidental language as those with normal hearing so parents should be told to incorporate activities that involve the use of mathematical expressions.

Visiting grandma, preparing for a visitor, cooking, shopping for new shoes, and endless other routine activities can be discussed with as much detail as the supermarket outing until parents learn how to make them real opportunities for learning language.

Feedback from one mother recently summed this up well when she said,

> "I tried what you said to do when going to the supermarket and I just couldn't believe how much we both enjoyed it. When we came home everybody who came into the house after that for two days had to hear about it! It takes much longer but it is so worthwhile."

The atmosphere in a parent guidance session should encourage parents to feel free to ask questions and, if necessary, express anxieties. At the same time, the guidance should result in their recognizing and looking for all the little progressions that can be identified. Parents and children should enjoy the sessions and should leave with a feeling of success.

Report on the Guidance Session

Immediately after the parent and child leave, a report of the session should be written. If the session was videotaped, it helps to review the tape as the report is being written. Points that have been missed during the live session can often be observed on the tape.

See Appendix B for a sample form that guides the way in which a session can be recorded. This report should be referred to as the basis on which the next session is planned.

Keep in mind that time should be left between parent guidance sessions to allow time for the report form on the preceding session to be filled out.

CHAPTER 5

Lessons Learned Worldwide From Observation of Interaction of Adults With Children Who Have a Hearing Loss

> "We consider that hearing children are usually in an ideal language learning situation and that these are exactly the conditions which must be provided for a hearing impaired child if he is going to use language confidently."
>
> (Wood et al., 1986)

Over the course of 20 years of international work, it has been possible to collect many samples of adults (parents and professionals) interacting with hearing-impaired children. Only those samples of adults who claimed to be following a "natural auditory oral approach" and so providing the conditions that Wood mentions above have been looked at in detail for this chapter. The aim has been to determine if the hearing-impaired children, with whom these adults were interacting, were indeed having the "same opportunity" as children with normal hearing would have at a similar language learning stage. In some cases they were, but in a large number of cases the linguistic opportunities occurring during the interaction were not the same as those that might be found in the case of a child with normal hearing. Only 63 of the 300 conversations analyzed could be classed as "natural." The lack of age-appropriate responses from the child with hearing loss often caused the adult to become more controlling and more vocabulary-centered than normal. The adults were usually unaware that they were interacting differently with the hearing-impaired child. The author has found it beneficial to use videotape excerpts to discuss this interaction with adults. Interestingly, most adults could identify the abnormalities independently when they had the opportunity to watch themselves on the videotapes. Almost all were surprised to find such differences from normal behavior. When these were addressed, the quality of interaction improved immediately so it seems important to highlight this area of our work.

In many situations where the author is called on to help a Natural Auditory Oral program develop, there is a basic need to help both parents and professionals distinguish between what can be considered "normal" age-appropriate, interactive behavior on their part and what cannot. There is no doubt the abnormalities exist because of the presence of hearing loss in the child. Another way of describing this problem is to look at what hearing loss does to the adults interacting with hearing-impaired children, as much as what it does to the children.

When attempting to decide what is and what is not "natural" or "normal," many aspects of an interaction must be observed. In this chapter, an attempt (based on the analysis of videotaped excerpts) is made to analyze some of the most important features that affect the normalcy of the interaction, so that those who are anxious to adopt a truly natural auditory oral approach can have guidelines. These can be summarized under the following headings:

1. Selection of material
2. Atmosphere in which interaction takes place
3. The nature of a conversation
4. Time to allow development of communicative behavior before first words are heard

5. Adequate provision of meaningful repetition
6. Use of normal, natural language in an interesting voice
7. Maintenance of the interaction
8. Sufficient experience of the seven functions of language
9. Constant testing of the child instead of conversation
10. Opportunities for repair.

Over the course of training professionals around the world, time and again a statement of the following type is made by someone anxious to change, "I'm much more comfortable working with the child myself than observing the parent because I know what to show them, but I don't really know what to say to parents after I've observed their interaction during a parent guidance session. Please give me an outline of what to do." In most cases, these professionals want some kind of a recipe or checklist that they can follow. It is important to address this situation, because the lack of confidence that it shows is one of the major reasons for not adopting the Natural Auditory Oral approach.

Each family is unique and every case is different. Professionals need to be capable of identifying any behavior in the interaction between adult and child that would not occur if the child had normal hearing. The many examples in this chapter are taken from different countries and different cultures. They illustrate how common the problems are worldwide. At the same time, discussion of them with the adults concerned has helped many to see the situation in a really practical light and to develop the confidence necessary for them to make a change to a much higher quality of interaction.

The Material

The way in which the topic or material used in the interaction is selected often determines all that follows. Factors to be considered are:

■ **Is the material age-appropriate?**
One interaction between an 11-year-old boy and a teacher failed because the boy lacked interest. It was little wonder as the material presented to the boy was a book about "The Three Bears." This is considered suitable material for preschool children but, when challenged, the teacher explained

very sincerely that this boy's language was not even at the level of a three-year-old. No matter how delayed the language of the child, the material used must be age-appropriate.

In contrast, a very normal interaction took place with an 11-year-old boy who was diagnosed very late, and whose expressive language was merely at the three-word level. He was encouraged to find a picture in a newspaper for each day's individual conversation and bring one from home every day. On the day he was observed, he communicated freely about Madonna and her guitar. All the prespeech behavior had had time to develop. He was motivated to share his ideas and was making his contributions in short phrases with real confidence. The therapist's behavior was interesting. She had established an excellent rapport with the boy and her main role was to encourage him. She gave her opinion about Madonna and the boy responded to her input, showing that he could take account of his conversational partner's contribution. This is the essence of a conversation.

■ **Does the child have any choice in the selection?**
Younger children, too, often respond quickly if offered choice in the subject or material to be discussed; for example, several books may be offered for them to choose the one they want or they may be given the choice of play dough or building blocks and so forth.

■ **Does the material hold the child's interest once the interaction has begun?**
All too often the interaction fades out after very few turns. Adults need to observe which topics motivate the child to interact with them and to plan material around these topics in the early stages of interacting with the child.

■ **Is the position in which the adult and child are placed, suitable for the material selected?**
In an abnormal number of observations children had to sit at tables. In several of the excerpts studied the interaction should have taken place on the floor and the child should have had the freedom that would allow natural control of the material in play, for example, when the material was a box of cars.

■ **Is the material to be used always supplied by the professional?**

Many teachers who give all guidance sessions in the children's homes have an "early support bag" that goes with them from house to house. No doubt it is full of interesting materials which the child does not have at home, and it catches the child's interest. However, when the professional leaves, parents must interact with the child through the everyday situation of the home. A balance must be kept between opportunities that the home provides naturally and those that are introduced by the professional, always bearing in mind that the routine situations of the home are there to be exploited linguistically and on a daily basis.

The Atmosphere in Which Communication Takes Place

It is important for professionals to understand the anxiety that can develop when parents come to realize the possibility and implications of the language delay associated with hearing loss in a young child. Often a sense of urgency drives parents to adopt a manner that has a negative effect on communication. The introduction of neonatal hearing screening is helping this picture to change. When children are fitted very early with appropriate amplification, it is easier for parents to believe that their child can learn to listen and talk following the normal pattern of language learning in any young child. This occurs because their listening skills are developing at around the normal age and therefore their responses are more normal. At this stage there need not be such a fear of serious delay.

Unfortunately, all too many children have their hearing loss diagnosed late. By this time, parents are very aware of the gap between the language skills of their children and those the same age with normal hearing. They are looking for shortcuts and often neglect the basic necessities of the early language learning process.

■ One primary task of those working with families who have a newly diagnosed child is to help them create an environment, at any age, in which the child will be motivated to learn language through age-appropriate activities and the routine of normal daily living, rather than setting out to teach the child language.

■ There were wide differences in the atmosphere in which communication took place. Where a relaxed atmosphere was created from the start, there was, without doubt, more normality.

The Nature of a Conversation

If a true conversation is to take place it is important to remember the old saying,

"Conversations cannot be planned, they happen."

At the same time it is important to remember that, although there is a definite structure to a conversation, this structure is not taught to children. It develops as they have opportunities to practice the skill of talking in conversational situations.

Conversation is so much a part of our daily lives that we give it little thought but, when we do think about it, we realize that:

■ Somehow we learn how to begin a conversation, to keep it going through its middle stages, and to draw it to a close.
■ People in a conversation take turns speaking.
■ Listeners in a conversation are not passive. If the conversation is to be successful there must be joint attention between the speaker and the listener.
■ Listeners often give nonverbal feedback to the speaker by nodding, shaking the head, and so forth.
■ Meaning in a conversation is often conveyed by prosody (pauses, rhythm, intonation, rate of utterance, accent), which helps the listener to understand, while at the same time giving the interaction a normal, local flavor.
■ There is no careful preplanning of the way a topic of a conversation should develop. Each move in a conversation is a reaction to the previous one.
■ Conversations do not always flow smoothly. It is quite normal and acceptable to find hesitations or false starts.
■ Misunderstandings often occur as conversations move along, but speakers who regularly engage in them learn how to repair such breakdowns.

■ Each turn in a conversation need not be a full sentence—
many are not. In several of the videotape excerpts children
were being made to answer in sentences when these were
not conversationally appropriate. For example, a child with
hearing loss who was asked his name, replied "Michael."
Immediately, the therapist with whom he was working said,
"Say that properly for me," and the child then replied, "My
name is Michael." This is quite unnatural in a conversational
situation and it marks a child as different. When this practice was questioned, the author was told that children with
hearing loss must learn to speak in sentences.

How do we learn all these things about conversations? No one
teaches a child a list of such "rules." Children come to them as they
have the opportunity to take part in conversations. For children with
hearing loss, therefore, it is very important that adults with whom
they interact understand the need to chat with the children about
any interests and to discuss the ordinary things of everyday living.

Development of Communicative Behavior
Before the First Words Develop

Wood reminds us how important the development of communicative behavior at the preverbal stage is. "Recent studies have shown
how the emergence of a child's first words represents the culmina-
tion of a process of communication that begins at birth" (Wood,
Wood, Wood, Griffiths, & Howarth. 1986).

Age-appropriate play, handled in an informal way and centered
on home activities, lays the foundations of communication. Children
with normal hearing and those with severe and profound hearing
losses alike respond to adults who behave in many different ways.
This allows communication to develop.

Create Situations in Which Joint Attention and
Joint Activity Are Established

In one case, a 2-year-old girl was helping her mother make
pastries and looked up expectantly after putting each cupful of
flour in the bowl and nodded to her mother showing that she was

a partner in this activity. This illustrates the development of preverbal communication.

In contrast, a two-year-old child and mother were playing with a bus and a box with little people in it. In this case, the mother aimed to teach the child to say, "in the bus" by showing her that people must go in the bus. But the child wanted to push the bus backward and forward and had no interest in the people. There was no joint attention throughout the activity, but rather a power struggle. Had the mother dropped her idea of filling the bus with people and started pushing the bus back and forth with the child, a very different language activity would have developed. There would have been lots of repetitive language, joint attention, and joint activity.

These examples show how necessary it is to observe communication between mother and child to see what is really happening. In both cases, the mother has set aside time to play with the child and was talking to the child; however, the second example illustrates clearly that acting with the same object does not automatically ensure that partners are talking about the same subject (Batliner, 2004).

Become Partners in the Child's Play

Play is work for young children and it is the means by which they come to terms with their environment. True play is initiated by the child, but at times, adults can become partners, and then both child and adult interact as they enjoy the activity. However, in many of the videotapes reviewed, problems were observed because adults often interrupted a child's play and began to organize it with the aim of "testing the child" or "teaching language."

In one example, a 5-year-old boy (C) with a cochlear implant was playing happily on the floor with a car track. He was making appropriate car noises and bumping the cars into each other. Mother (M) intervened as follows:

M: (Holding up a motorbike) Look, What's this?

C: No response—continues to play bumper cars.

M: What is it? Look here.

C: No response.

M: (Taking one car away from the child and holding up the motorbike). Look at this one. What is it?

C: Child shrugs and tries to take back his car.

M: (To author) He's a naughty boy. He knows what it is but just won't say it.
(To child) It's a motorbike. You know that, say "motorbike."

C: Motorbike.

The child's play was completely disrupted by this exchange, and as a result, he had no desire to communicate with his mother nor to include her in his play. Her intervention was completely unproductive. She felt like a failure and was annoyed with the child.

Parents must learn to follow rather than direct the child in the early stages of communication and particularly in play situations. When this happens, the child is provided with language in context and gradually comes to make sense of the language from the contextual cues.

Adults must also be aware that children are not really interested in the names of things, but rather in what things can do and what they can do with them. It is usually active situations that motivate young children to attend, to learn to listen, and to use language. Parents and professionals must be led to understand the importance of determining what is holding the child's interest and to use that as the basis for conversation.

Most young children enjoy playing with a ball. They will be in a good language-learning situation if the word "ball" is used in context instead of being "taught" formally that, "This is a ball." Phrases and sentences referring to action with the ball offer natural repetition and are what will eventually lead to the child's understanding of the concept, For example:

- Roll the ball.
- Catch the ball.
- Oh, you dropped the ball.
- Here's a bigger ball.

Tassoni and Hucker (2000) emphasize very strongly how much children learn from firsthand experiences provided in play. The skill of the adult in play situations is to interact in such a way that the child feels comfortable and is happy to have the adult contributing to and extending the play.

Regulate Turn Taking

Referring to the language development of children with normal hearing, Snow (1977) feels that the main purpose of adults' conversations with young children seems to be to encourage the children to take turns. The importance of turn-taking cannot be overestimated because no real conversation can take place unless it exists.

Without thinking about it, parents talking to young children adopt certain strategies that help the development of turn taking.

Recognition of the Child's Communicative Attempts

Recognition of any communicative attempt by a child is an important feature in the development of turn taking. Parents can be observed responding even to behavior that is not intentionally communicative on the part of the child, for example,

A baby yawns

Mother immediately says," Oh you are so sleepy"

Baby yawns again

Mother, "Yes, you are sleepy."

Although there is no deliberate turn-taking by the child, reactions of this kind by an adult give the impression that a dialogue is taking place. This is extremely important as it indicates a stage in the early linguistic development that is common to all children learning language.

As children grow more communicative their first moves may well be nonverbal, for example, pointing, smiling appropriately, and so on. Gradually, these early nonverbal responses grow into verbal turns. The emotional atmosphere in which these contributions are received is very important. The verbal response of the adult may take many forms:

- Merely a sustaining move like "Oh" or "Mm"

- An imitation of the child's contribution
    Child: "Home"
    Mother: "Oh, home"

- An expansion of what child says
    Child: "Daddy, work"
    Mother: " Yes, Daddy's still at work"

The addition of "Yes" may seem unimportant, but it does in fact help to create the desired warm atmosphere, because it carries with it the assurance to the child that his idea was right and has been understood. In her work with children in Germany who are hearing impaired, Batliner (2004) found that, just as parents of children with normal hearing are always unconsciously one step ahead of the child in their linguistic level, parents of children with a hearing loss develop in the same way once they become confident in their ability to communicate with their child.

Use of the Pause

In many of the excerpts of videotape analyzed, the adults talked so much that there was no opportunity for the child to make a communicative move. Carey-Sargeant and Brown (2003) highlight the important role of the pause in interaction between mother and young child in the early stages of language development.

Two contrasting styles of interaction illustrate this well. In the first example, a mother with a newly diagnosed $2^1/_2$ year-old with a profound hearing loss was so aware of the little girl's need for language that she talked incessantly, completely ignoring the child's early need for communicative behavior to be allowed to develop.

M: Look we're going to clean these dirty shoes

C: Child puts out a hand to take a shoe

M: No, no. Look how dirty they are first. Look it's all muddy here. We need to wash off the mud first and then we'll use this polish. They'll be nice and clean then. You like clean shoes don't you?

C: Child begins to lose interest

M: Look here. This is the cloth and we'll wet it (takes the child by the hand to the sink). This is where the water comes from to wet the cloth. I'll turn on the tap and you'll see the water. Look here it comes. Now our cloth is wet.

This was a very appropriate activity and the mother really wanted to involve the child. She was aware when the child's interest began to decrease and took her by the hand, but continued to talk so much that there was no pause for a verbal or nonverbal response from the child and so a basic communicative skill had no chance to emerge. Contrast that with the interaction of another mother and child of a similar age engaged in the same activity.

M: Look how dirty your shoes are

C: (Time given to child to look at the shoes). Child gestures with a brushing movement

M: That's right we need to brush them. Where's the brush? (mother looks around)

C: Child points to a cupboard

M: Let's take the brush out

C: Nods and runs to the cupboard

M: (Brushing a shoe.) I'll brush this one and you brush that one.

C: Child vocalizes as he brushes and then holds his shoe up for approval.

M: Oh, what a good job you've done.

The pace of this interaction allowed for normal pausing, which is an important feature of conversational behavior. An experienced conversational partner realizes immediately when it is time to take a turn. For a child in the early stages of linguistic development, however, the pause may have to be extended a little to indicate to the child that a response is expected. In many of the observations made, the linguistic retardation caused by the hearing loss seemed to result in slower responses from a child with a hearing loss and, in a conversation, the pause was often longer. Some adults then rushed in to fill the silence and thus denied the child the opportunity to take a turn. Other adults left too long a pause, resulting in both partners becoming uncomfortable.

It is important to take note of this linguistic feature because, when the pause is a comfortable length, it leads to:

- An opportunity for a child to take a turn and possibly to frame an answer to a question
- Freedom for the child to initiate a new move in a conversation
- Spontaneous imitation of what has been offered by the adult

Acknowledgment of Imitation

In interactions between adults and young children, whether with normal hearing or with a hearing loss, one of the strategies adopted by the children at the language learning stage is that of imitation, for example, an adult and 3-year-old child with a cochlear implant are looking at a book.

A: What's happening in this picture?

C: Fire in house.

A: Yes, there's a fire in that house.

C: A fire in that house.

A: What are these people doing?

C: Looking fire.

A: That's right, listen. They're looking at the fire

C: Looking at the fire.

A: I think that they'll phone the Fire brigade, what do you think?

C: Talk the phone.

A: Yes, I think they'll talk on the phone

C: Talk on the phone.

A: Who will they phone?

C: Fire people.

A: Yes we call these people firemen

C: Firemen.

Where attention has been paid to the place of imitation in early language development several interesting observations have been made:

- Imitation happens by both partners in a conversation—child imitates adult and adult "imitates" child. This shows the child that what was said was heard, was accepted, and was put into a conventional spoken language pattern.
- Children have been found to imitate spontaneously mainly words or grammatical structures that are not at that time part of their stable vocabulary or language system and to stop the imitation once these have become part of it (Crystal, 1997).
- Imitation is one of the many features of interaction closely interwoven with other key elements (joint attention, joint activity, etc.) in the developing language of a child.
- It has a special place in the development of the language of a child with a hearing loss because adults can learn so much by listening to the imitation. It provides:
  - Evidence of the child's level of listening
  - The current length of utterance
  - The use of prosodic means (intonation, loudness, rhythm) in the child's speech
  - The ability of the child to receive and begin to make spontaneous linguistic offerings of his own.

Not all children with a hearing loss come to this stage spontaneously and there are certain unobtrusive strategies that adults can use to lead them into it:

- Turning to the child with an expectant expression
- Before the adult offers an expansion, a simple prompt like, "listen" may be given

At the same time care must be taken not to:

- Ask the child deliberately to repeat what has been said, because this often leads to meaningless repetition
- "Overwork" on an attempted imitation to perfect it, because in that way the flow of interaction is disrupted
- Give negative feedback about the child's imperfect imitation because this can cause the child to lose confidence and to become reluctant to try further spontaneous imitations

Adequate Provision of Meaningful Repetition

The normal routine of a home provides many opportunities for natural repetition. In most homes, the same things happen at the same time daily from Monday to Friday. This regularity provides opportunities for the reinforcement of language in a familiar situation, for example, the collecting of clothes to be washed. These can be sorted by color or by material and as they are put into the washing machine or the sink there can be meaningful chatter about each item. One such session went like this

M: (Holding a bag full of washing) Oh, what a lot of washing we have today.

C: Pull.

M: That's right, pull it out. What a big shirt Daddy has.

C: Pull.

M: Yes, we'll pull another one out.

C: Not Daddy.

M: No, it's not Daddy's shirt. That's Frank's shirt (points to photo of Frank on the wall). Pull out another one.

C: No more.

M: You're right, there are no more shirts. Pull something else out now.

And so the talk went on as the activity progressed. This mother and little boy were wholly in tune with each other. His imperfect utterances were fully understood by the mother who kept the activity going while, at the same time, reinforcing and extending the language as the occasion arose.

This type of experience arises in many home situations and it is important for parents to realize what valuable language learning opportunities these situations present. One mother who had transferred from a very formal program said, "I enjoy every minute I spend with her now and can't believe that she is learning so much without my teaching anything!"

Wells (1979), who studied children at the language-learning stage in their homes, found that children usually initiated the verbal interactions. They tried to talk about what they were doing or interested in and parents joined in. As we observe parents interacting with a child who has a hearing loss, this is one area to watch for and help to develop because all too often the parents feel the need to start the interaction on every occasion.

Use of Normal Natural Language with an Interesting Voice

It was surprising to find how many adults in the video excerpts used an almost telegraphic form of speech instead of fluent language. This destroyed the features of rhythm, intonation, and accent (prosody) that adults use with young children with normal hearing. In such a situation, the child with a hearing loss is deprived of the natural input on which the intelligibility of our spoken language depends.

For example, one mother was making a sandwich with a boy with a profound hearing loss, aged three years, four months. She spoke in such a way as to destroy the rhythm and intonation of the language:

M: (Taking material out of a basket) Look—bread, butter, knife, jam, plate.

C: Picks up knife.

M: (Pulling at the knife) No—dangerous—might cut

C: Struggles for the knife.

M: (With knife in her hand, pointing to the bread) Spread what?

C: Points to jam.

M: No, first butter.

Another mother, who was asked to make a sandwich with a boy of 3 years, 5 months with a profound hearing loss, provided a very different linguistic experience in a very natural voice:

M: (Holding out a plastic bag full of materials for the sandwich) Come and have a look at what I have here.

C: Takes out the bread and the plate.

M: Good boy, put the bread on the plate. (Pauses while child does this) Now, what should we do? (Waits)

C: Takes out the knife and the jam.

M: (Holds up the butter) Don't you want this first?

C: Shakes head and touches the jam.

M: Oh, all right, that's fine.

This mother was supplying the child with a wealth of normal, natural language with all the melodic features of English. It is interesting too that, even at this early stage, the mother allowed for choice. It was not at all important whether the butter or jam went on the bread. The mother respected the child's choice.

In such a relaxed atmosphere mother and child become partners and enjoy the interaction. This mother has learned to talk "with," not "at," the child and in so doing she uses the interesting voice that mothers use when communicating with young children.

Maintenance of the Interaction

Normal conversations involve a number of turns on the part of the communicating partners. In conversations with very young children or even older children in the case of the hearing impaired, it is often difficult to keep the communication flowing. At the early stages, the responsibility for this rests on the shoulders of the adult partner. Once again certain strategies can be identified but, as in the case of other strategies, the adult is not always conscious of their use. Mothers in particular provide a "language acquisition support system for their children" (Bruner, 1983) all unconsciously, and part of this is their ability to keep the interaction flowing in a variety of ways. Unfortunately, in the presence of a hearing loss in the child, the provision of this support system is often absent. It consists of several different elements.

Expansion

It is common for adults to expand a child's contribution as in the following dialogue between a mother and her four-year-old girl who has had a cochlear implant for two years.

C: Tomorrow go to zoo?

M: Yes, we'll go to the zoo tomorrow.

C: See elephants?

M: I hope we'll see elephants. They're very big.

C: (Stretching out hands) Big like this?

M: Oh, much bigger than that.

In that short dialogue, two kinds of expansion can be found.

1. A simple expansion to make part of it grammatically correct, "Yes, we'll go to the zoo."
2. An addition to the topic in the form of talk about the size of elephants.

Statements

A further idea, in the form of a statement related to the topic, may be added as a means of keeping the conversation going or of offering an explanation.

M: I think we'll see polar bears at the zoo, too.

C: Oh, white ones?

M: Yes, white furry ones.

C: What for furry?

M: They live where it is very cold and the fur keeps them warm.

C: At home, fur on my hands.

M: That's right. You have gloves with fur on them to keep your hands warm.

Questions

Questions can be a real means of maintaining the interaction through directing the attention of the children in a way that will motivate them to make further contributions to the dialogue. Care needs to be taken, however, to make sure that they do not dominate the dialogue and that they are not merely a way of testing the child.

There are many varieties of question form and it is important that the questions asked should be matched to the interest and linguistic level of the children. Basically there are closed and open questions. The closed questions require, on the whole, only one-word answers and are not so likely to maintain the dialogue. The type of question used determines to a certain extent, the type of linguistic experience offered to the child; 78% of the questions asked in the interactions recorded for this study were closed questions requiring only one-word answers.

Open questions, on the other hand, bring with them a freedom that offers a child the opportunity to express his or her opinion in other than just a single word. Adults sometimes feel less secure with open questions because they cannot always predict the answer and cannot always understand the child. It is often necessary to remind parents of children with a hearing loss that parents of children with normal hearing experience the same kind of frustration when the child is at the early language learning stage.

Initially the adult may have to play a double part by answering as well as asking the question so that the child becomes familiar with the questioning situation. This may lead to a situation in which a limited choice is given and the child merely has to identify one of two alternatives, for example:

Why did the farmer make holes there?

No response.

Did he want to fill them with water or to put plants in them?

Put plants in.

Children develop confidence in such situations and learn that they are responsible for giving a response. It is important, though, not to let this stage go on for too long because children can get into the habit of waiting for the choice and not making enough effort to think of the answer independently.

One difficulty lies in the fact that, in normal life, in a true dialogue, questions are asked only when one conversational partner does not know the answer. Young children with a hearing loss are often bombarded with questions that, by no means, always lead to the maintenance of a conversation. One reason for this is the need of the adult to get the child to say something. This, in turn, often leads to irrelevant closed questions to which the child knows that the adult knows the answer, for example, when a child is describing a situation in a picture, the adult feels the dialogue coming to a close and tries to extend it by asking meaninglessly what color things are or how many there are of them. This in fact creates a test situation rather than a conversational one. For example as one adult was sharing a book with a child, what started out as a good conversational situation turned into a test.

A: What is the farmer doing?

C: Get milk cow.

A: That's right, he's milking the cow.
     What else is happening?

C: No response.

Failing to sustain the topic, the adult then changed to a test situation in which success would be ensured:

A: Look! How many cows are there?

C: Three.

A: What color are they?

C: Brown.

In this situation, the adult's need to feel that the conversation had been successful led to the use of completely irrelevant questions and lowered the linguistic level of what started out as a good conversation to a mere test.

Children as Agents in Maintaining the Interaction

It is now appropriate to turn attention to observations of the part that children who are hearing impaired may play in maintaining the flow of conversations. The behavior of the child has a significant effect on the adult conversational partner. Much of the abnormal behavior of the adults observed can be attributed to the lack of normal age-appropriate responses from the child.

Any acknowledgement on the part of the child of the adult's contribution serves to keep the interaction flowing because it raises awareness in the adult that the child is an active partner in the conversation. These child acknowledgements may take many forms, for example, very normal nonverbal turn, such as an interested facial expression or nodding or a verbal turn, such as:

- A single word
- A question
- A statement.

Experience of the Reasons for Which We Use Language

It is important to bear in mind the various reasons for which we use language and to expose hearing-impaired children to statements and questions that will encourage their use. Tough (1977) lists seven functions as:

- **Self-maintenance**
  A: Why did you do that?
  C: I didn't do it. It was John.

■ **Directing**

A: Stick the white paper on the corner.

C: It should go there.

■ **Reporting**

A: What did you do at the camp?

C: Slept in a big tent—very cold.

■ **Reasoning**

A: How do you know that it's not a math lesson?

C: Because the children are painting and making models. They do that in art.

■ **Predicting**

A: What do you think will happen next?

C: The boy will fall in the water and the man will jump in to save him.

■ **Projecting**

A: How do you think he felt about that?

C: He was very happy.

■ **Imagining**

A: How do you think the story ended?

C: A fairy came and gave all the children a present.

Care must be taken not to ask too many questions that lead merely to the reporting function. Over 85% of the questions asked in the videotapes studied provided the child with the opportunity to report something. In the traditional oral approach to the education of children with a hearing loss, this function was very much overemphasized with the result that there was little opportunity for children to practice using language across a range of functions. Even today, parents are often surprised when they are advised to encourage their young child with a hearing loss to think what might happen next or to describe how someone might feel. Recently, the author was asked by a parent, "But isn't that too difficult for him to do since he's deaf?" Students, too, often express surprise when observing a teacher with high expectations in relation to the functions of language to which she exposes the children. In the past, ceilings of expectation were often set by professionals or parents. Consequently, children with a hearing loss had reduced experience of language at the vital language learning stage.

Instances can be found where children with a hearing loss, at different levels of communicative competence, use strategies to enlarge on or further maintain the interaction. For example:

- Relating to his own experience—one little boy (4 years, 3 months old) commented on the weather at his home, when looking at a snowy picture. The therapist asked questions about the snow.
- Pointing to move the story on—in the same conversation, when this little boy had said all he wanted to say about the snow at home, he pointed to the next part of the story that he wanted to discuss saying, "Look."

Temptation to Assess the Child Constantly

Another reason for too many questions arising in a conversation may be a "teacher attitude" on the part of the adult who wants to check that information previously learned has been remembered. Parents are often so anxious to show that their child with a hearing loss is making the progress that they so much long for that they ask questions to give themselves the satisfaction of hearing the child say something that they know he or she knows.

There was a strange case of a mother, father, and child coming into a parent guidance situation where the mother was very proud that the child could now say "Mama" and "Papa." She wanted to show this off to the professional and said to the child (totally out of context) "Say Mama!" The child smiled and mother repeated, "Say Mama!" with no response from the child. The mother then changed to "Say Papa!" with still no response from the child. Both parents were very disappointed and the father sitting next to the child went into his pocket to produce a photo of himself and said to the child "Look! Here's Papa! Say Papa!" The child looked at the professional and smiled. The professional brought this test to a close by saying, "I hear you're a clever boy now and can say Mama and Papa." This satisfied the parents.

Added to this abnormality is the possibility that, when the child does not respond with the required answer, the same question may be repeated up to six or even eight times in exactly the same words. This is very threatening to the child. If the answer is not given after the question has been asked twice in the same form, the wording should be changed and more information given to the child in the hope of leading him or her to the answer.

Care needs to be taken by those assessing the progress of children following cochlear implants. It is understandable that certain aspects of the child's progress, particularly those related to the use of hearing, need careful monitoring, but in some programs, children are subjected to up to three hours at a time of tests of linguistic progress and so forth. This is worrying for both parents and child.

Handling Conversational Repair

From time to time, misunderstandings occur in any conversation and the partners take steps to clear these up. This presents little difficulty where both partners are experienced users of the language. However, more difficulty arises when repair is needed and the partners' linguistic levels are uneven. When interacting with hearing-impaired children of a low linguistic level, some adults cope well and try to clear up the misunderstanding by showing something concrete, by questioning further, or by offering explanations at a simpler linguistic level. In other cases, however, the need for repair forces an adult to offer lengthy and involved explanations, far above the child's comprehension. Other adults, put off by the misunderstanding, are inclined to pass over it and move on without attempting repair. This can lead to further confusion.

Where conversations between adult and child are a regular feature of interaction in a relaxed atmosphere, it is interesting to find, not only the adult, but also the child developing the skill to recognize and address misunderstandings when they occur.

One six-year-old boy who had a cochlear implant for just over a year came into a regular class one Monday to give his news to his hearing friends. The conversation went like this:

C: On Sunday, I have two lambs in my home.

A: In the house?

C: No, not two in—really only one.

A: Where was the other?

C: In the field.

A: Why was that?

C: Not both babies. One was mother.

A: Oh, you had one lamb and one sheep.

C: Yes—baby in the house—Mummy in the field.

Other misunderstandings frequently arise when the topic changes. In many instances, a shift in topic can be identified in normal conversational situations. When children with hearing loss have ample opportunity to converse, we find that they are capable of moving off topic to relate to their own experience. For example, an eight-year-old boy with profound hearing loss was discussing a picture of a traffic accident in which there was a policeman. He suddenly said, "I be a policeman when I big" and the following dialogue ensued:

A: "You want to be a policeman?"

C: "Yes, I catch the thieves."

A: " What will you do with the thieves?"

C: "I put them in prison" (then returning to the picture he continued) This one not. This one car."

A: That's right that policeman is finding out what happened with the car.

Other children can be very confused when the adult tries to leave the actual picture in discussion and learn to cope in such situations only after repeated exposure to them. When children with hearing loss have ample opportunity for individual conversation sessions, they often to learn to cope with a shift. This allows the possibility for not only more turns in the conversation, but also for the opportunity to relate the topic to their own experience. On the other hand, hearing impaired children who do not have this experience are often very rigid and do not find it easy to change topics. As a result, the conversation comes to a more abrupt end or more concrete support is needed to help the child make the shift.

A: What is the girl, holding?

C: The window.

A: No, these are not a window. They go at the window. What do we call them?

C: Don't know.

A: They're curtains.

C: Oh.

A: You have curtains on your windows at home. Are they the same as these?

C: (pointing to the curtains in the picture) Curtains.

A: Yes, these are curtains. Tell me about your curtains at home.

C: No response.

It is important to build opportunities into the program that help children develop the ability to leave a topic so as to link the conversation with their own experience.

Hearing-impaired children can be sensitive to the need for repair in a conversational situation. For example, they may be aware that they and the adult are not understanding each other and may take the initiative in dealing with the situation. This represents a higher linguistic skill.

Sometimes the adult sees a confused look on the child's face, indicating that what has gone before was not understood. Other times, the child may repeat part of the adult's contribution with an intonation suggesting there is some doubt about what has been said. This provides an opportunity for the adult to elaborate. It is important for adults to provide children with the appropriate language opportunities in which to express misunderstandings.

Throughout this chapter, many conversational features have been addressed. According to the author's experience, these are important areas to explore when helping adults reach a higher quality of interaction with hearing-impaired children. As in all other skills, practice is the key to improving ability to share meaning in conversational sessions. The more frequent the interactions, the more confidence grows on the part of both adults and children who come to expect to, and do understand, each other. When this environment is achieved, there is a greater possibility that hearing-impaired children will have the same opportunity to develop language naturally as those with normal hearing.

CHAPTER 6

Educational Placement

> *"Inclusion has been acclaimed as a force for renewing schools and the route to building more inclusive and equitable societies."*
>
> **(Lim & Tan, 2004)**

This chapter is based on the author's personal experience in developing inclusion programs. However, it by no means covers the full variety of such programs worldwide. Wherever reference is made to a specific program, the corresponding country is mentioned. Several areas already covered in this book are considered in this chapter from a different angle.

When educational placement is considered for a child with a hearing impairment, it is important for parents and those responsible for placement to be fully aware of the range of available placement opportunities as well as the trend toward inclusion worldwide. Situations differ from one region to another, but over the years, placement options have come to include one or more of the following:

■ A special school
■ A unit for children with hearing loss placed in a mainstream school under the instruction of a qualified teacher for the deaf

- A group of children with hearing loss placed in a mainstream school with on-site or visiting teacher support
- A single child with hearing loss in a regular school, with or without support.

Recently, several variations of these options have been developed, and are outlined in this chapter.

Historically, only special schools were available to meet the needs of hearing-impaired children; many of those schools were boarding schools. Several factors combined to reduce the need for such establishments during the second half of the 20th century:

- Improved audiological techniques that led to more accurate and earlier diagnosis of deafness
- Provision of better acoustic signals to the children by constantly improving hearing aids
- The development of FM wireless communication
- The development of cochlear implants
- Children developing spoken language earlier than before thanks to parent guidance programs. As a result, parents want to keep the child in the family rather than accept placement in a residential school. This leads to greater parent involvement with professionals in the child's education.
- Changed public attitudes toward handicaps of any kind
- Official education acts recommending, and in some cases insisting, that wherever possible a child should be educated in his or her neighborhood school
- The development of support services by local education authorities with visiting teacher services.

Inclusion or Integration

Inclusion is a relatively new term, which grew out of an expanded integration concept. Both terms have as their ultimate aim the placement of a child with special needs in a mainstream setting. In practice, however, the two approaches are often very different.

In integration, a pupil with special needs may be placed in the school on the school's terms. The child is expected to adapt to the existing situation and curriculum. Depending on the location of the school, the child may or may not have support there. Parents often have a very heavy responsibility to help the child to keep pace with the curriculum.

Inclusion is the much wider concept of adapting the environment and the curriculum to suit the pupil with special needs. This represents mainstream education on the pupil's terms. The full adoption of the inclusion principle places a heavy responsibility on the professionals responsible for the child's placement. There needs to be a fundamental reappraisal of all educational activities to ensure that they are available to all children in the program.

Worldwide, inclusion of special needs children in regular classrooms is growing, but the quality of its provisions for the children varies greatly from one place to another. It is important to consider various models of inclusion. In this chapter, these models are outlined together so that readers may fully understand what is involved in the provision of quality education in an inclusion model.

Historical Background

If we are to understand the educational policies leading to today's demands for mainstream education for hearing-impaired children, it is necessary to trace the movements that have developed in various parts of the world. Their roots lie far back in history.

During the 19th century, as education for all became compulsory, deaf and blind children were the first children with disabilities to receive attention. Their disabilities were obvious and governments saw that proper education could lead to greater independence and job opportunities. In Britain and other European countries, special schools developed to cater to the special needs of children known at that time as deaf and blind. Initially, these were charitable institutions, but by the end of the 19th century, governments intervened and took responsibility for this education. Pritchard (1963) points out that, at the beginning of the 19th century, only 5% of deaf children received education of any kind. However, by the end of that century, the vast majority of deaf children were receiving full-time education in special schools for the deaf.

The foundations of today's movement toward inclusion of children who are hearing impaired in regular schools were being laid more than a hundred years ago. Within the special schools of the time, it became obvious that, in spite of their limited communication skills, hearing-impaired children had abilities. It was clear that they could become part of the general workforce, although for the most part they could find work only in occupations below their abilities. Lynas (1994) pointed out that, "The notion that schools for the deaf should prepare their pupils for life in wider society, rather than provide a means of escaping it, gained greater acceptance at this time."

During the 20th century, many factors combined to revolutionize opportunities for hearing-impaired children. Most important is the concept that these children have the capacity to learn what their normal hearing counterparts can learn, if the environment permits. This puts responsibility on those seeking to identify children's needs by including them in regular schools and making sure the environment really does permit each child to reach his or her full potential.

Knowledge of what causes hearing loss improved during the first half of the 20th century, as did knowledge of hearing mechanisms. Audiology developed as a science and provided a means of accurately measuring hearing loss. It soon became clear that the majority of children with hearing loss had useful residual hearing and only a tiny proportion, if any, was totally deaf.

In spite of these advances, only a limited number of people questioned the segregation of hearing-impaired children into special schools. The new English Education Act of 1944 was responsible for moving things forward. This Act allowed a child with an identified disability to attend an ordinary school. It caused the real movement toward inclusion to begin in the second half of the 20th century and it has gained momentum from that time on, not only in Britain, but worldwide.

The 21st Century

Definition of Need, Not of Handicap

Today, children are no longer classified according to a disability, but rather according to each child's individual needs arising from that disability and this provides the basis on which special help is supplied. Until recently, the medical model of disability, existed alone.

Today, it is gradually being replaced by a social model. In this model, people are recognized as full citizens who need to be accepted in inclusive educational programs.

In some countries, however, there has been, and still is, reluctance to include children with special needs in regular classes because of the fear that their presence would lower the overall standard of work. For example, there have been problems finding schools in Ecuador that are willing to include children with special needs. However, things are changing. For many years, several children from a private program for children with hearing loss have been included in private schools. It is encouraging to find that, recently, the Conocoto program, near Quito, which serves children who cannot afford private school fees, has forged links with a nearby primary school. This program is supporting the children and their parents, in the afternoons on a regular basis.

Two children are seen in Figure 6–1 receiving support from the coordinator of the special school program who has good contact with the school in which they are placed.

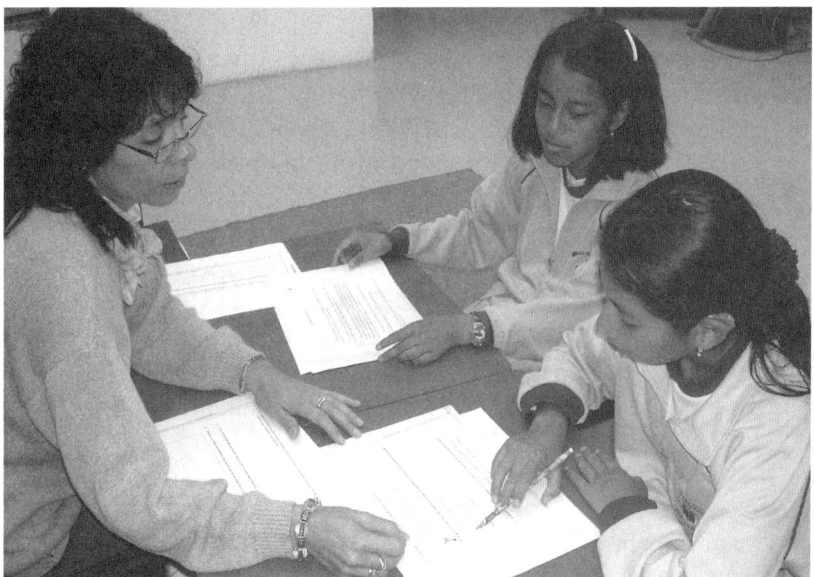

Figure 6–1. *Therapist supporting the work of two pupils included in a regular Ecuadorian school. (One has a profound hearing loss and the other a severe hearing loss.)*

There is no such thing as the "typical hearing-impaired child" and, therefore, there is no simple blueprint for programs of inclusion. The specific educational needs of each child must be taken into account when placing the child into the best educational environment to suit his or her needs. This places big demands on those responsible for providing support services for children with hearing loss.

In inclusive education, parents and class teachers in mainstream schools are in constant contact with the hearing-impaired child and must be empowered to deal with the special needs of that child. These "ordinary" teachers and parents spend the most time with the children and they must become both confident and competent in meeting the special needs of any child for whose education they are responsible. This realization represents a shift away from the belief that only "experts" in the field of a special disability can help the child with his or her problem. It requires professionals to be committed to empowering parents and classroom teachers in mainstream schools so that they become capable of devising the curriculum and approaches to meet the needs of all their pupils. It is interesting to discover an extension of good practice for all the children in a class when thought is given to the specific needs of a particular child. An outstanding example of this is a mainstream program in Pretoria, South Africa in which 20% of the children are hearing impaired. Parents of children with normal hearing are constantly remarking on the improved linguistic skills of their children.

Those who organize support services need to make sure they are always aware of new developments in the special needs fields for which they are responsible. One example of this is the necessity for frequency modulation (FM) systems in regular classrooms for children with impaired hearing (Figure 6-2). These are linked to the pupils' personal hearing aids with three main advantages. They:

■ Cut the distance between the teacher and the child
■ Reduce the effect of reverberation
■ Cut out the background noise.

The clear FM signal that reaches the child's ear is a major benefit in a regular classroom.

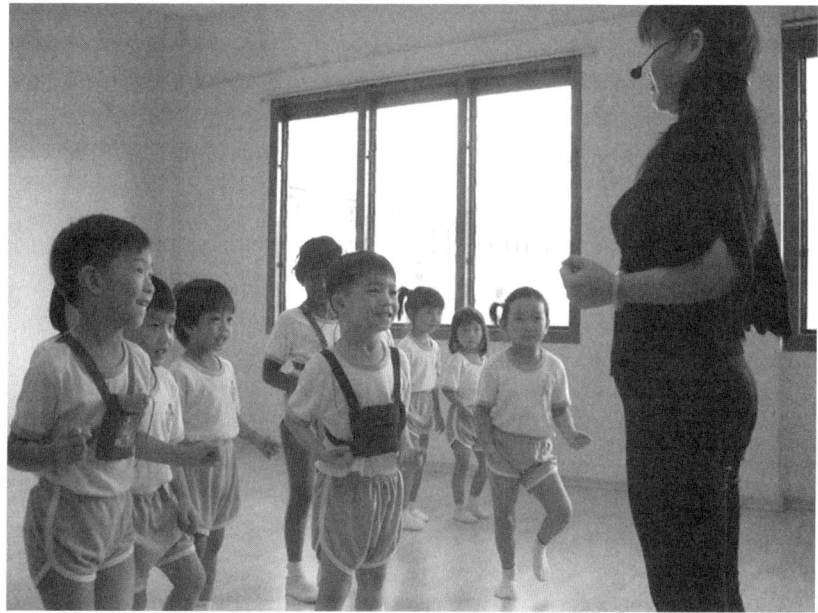

Figure 6–2. *Children who are hearing impaired benefit from the use of an FM system in a Singapore music and movement class.*

If the support teachers come from special schools operating in the past, they must have high enough expectations for today's children who are hearing impaired. Supported by good parent guidance, the lives of today's young children with a hearing loss are being revolutionized by what can be achieved, even at the pre-school stage. Very early diagnosis, combined with early issuance of appropriate amplification through hearing aids or cochlear implants, as well as parent guidance programs that help parents manage their child independently, can lead to a spoken language learning pattern similar to that of a child with normal hearing.

In addition, it is necessary to remember that not every pupil will be placed in the most appropriate mainstream school. When the definition of inclusion suggests that the education of pupils with special needs should take place in "appropriate settings," this does not necessarily mean exclusively in mainstream schools. For certain pupils with very special needs, special schools may indeed be the places where their needs are best met.

In many areas, children of secondary school age experience severe difficulties in inclusive situations, mainly because they lack appropriate support. They may not reach the academic levels they are capable of. Mary Hare Grammar School in England, which operates on a wholly auditory/oral approach, caters specifically to hearing-impaired children who are academically able. The pupils there reach a high academic level and many of them go on to full university courses.

It is important to realize that placement in a special school does not necessarily imply the school has a signing program. For many years, the author was principal of a large special school for children with severe and profound hearing loss in which no signs were used in or out of class. Spoken language was the mode of communication throughout and, on leaving school, the students were able to fit comfortably into society at large. They were even able go on to a higher education program designed for children with normal hearing.

The author is currently acting as an international advisor on the education of children with hearing impairment in 12 countries and, as such, sees many different patterns of inclusion in action. Different cultures and societies have different needs, but there are certain basic areas of need that form the foundation of any efficient support service. These needs vary with different ages and educational stages.

The Preschool Stage

Audiological Management

By the time children with hearing impairment enter an educational program, their parents or caregivers should have attended a parent guidance program in which they learn about the use and management of the hearing instruments worn by the child. They must ensure that the child enjoys daylong listening. Thus, for pupils with hearing impairment, consideration must be given to support services at the preschool stage.

The support must be given by audiologists who are knowledgeable about today's test procedures and the range of hearing instruments available and have the ability to fit appropriate instruments efficiently and provide reliable maintenance of them.

The foundations for successful inclusion are laid at the pre-school stage. It is sad that, in some countries where the economic situation is poor, it is a luxury to consider provision of services for children below compulsory school age.

The staff of regular kindergarten programs need to be counseled before children with a hearing loss are placed there. Careful monitoring of the children's progress needs to be arranged as well. This information should not be restricted to the child's classroom teacher. Others involved in special areas of the curriculum also need to be made fully aware of a child's needs, for example, the need for FM in music and movement sessions.

Linguistic Development

Even today, many children born with hearing impairment miss the spoken language element of the early home environment because their hearing loss is diagnosed late. As a result, when fitted with appropriate amplification (hearing aids or cochlear implants), they are late in learning to listen and in developing communicative behavior. Amplification alone does not compensate for hearing loss. Parents must learn how important it is to speak with the child about all the daily occurrences in the family. In addition, as reported in Chapter 5, parents who become anxious about lack of normal responses from a young hearing-impaired child often begin to communicate with the child in a way that is far from providing the same opportunity as a child with normal hearing would have. They need help as soon as possible to give this child the same opportunities as a child with normal hearing. This is vital preparation for inclusion in a mainstream school.

In the parent guidance program, parents should come to the realization that a mother tongue is "caught" not "taught" and that communicative behavior develops before spoken language. They can then be led to realize that the normal routine of the home provides a valuable language-enabling environment in preparation for inclusive education.

Most children with normal hearing enter school able to understand what is said to them and to express themselves in fluent, spoken language. School teaches them, for the most part, through the medium of spoken language and they are expected to communicate in and out of class in spoken language.

The importance of a child's development in spoken language cannot be overemphasized. For example, Robertson and Flexer (2000) provide evidence of a high correlation between fluency of spoken language and competence in literacy. This will, in time, give the pupil independent access to study material.

In the United Kingdom, the majority of hearing-impaired children are placed in regular kindergartens with support from visiting teachers of the deaf. The frequency of visits from the specialist teachers depends on the linguistic and educational level of the child. Many teachers visit once a week or more. Sometimes the visiting teacher alternates between visits to the kindergarten and visits to the home. This allows those who interact with the child in the preschool situation to be trained while parents are steadily guided along.

Since the late 1980s, the Canossian School in Singapore has run a program in which parents participate in individual guidance sessions. There is no fixed syllabus that every family must follow because advice is given on an "observation model" and guidance is unique to the particular needs of each family. This begins immediately after diagnosis and continues at least until children reach primary school age.

When a child in this program reaches nursery school or kindergarten, arrangements are made for admission to an included program of the appropriate age level. Children with hearing loss spend at least one more hour per day in their program than their peers with normal hearing. This allows children to prepare for their lessons and study the language that will be used the following day as well as to review what has been covered that day. It keeps children from missing new material because they have to be taken out of the mainstream class while subjects are taught to the rest of the class.

In the Eduplex in Pretoria, South Africa, the first fully inclusionary program, in that country, for children with hearing loss began in 2002. Twenty percent of the normal kindergarten class is comprised of hearing-impaired children. Play provides excellent opportunities for inclusion and children with hearing loss grow socially in play situations (see Figure 6-3).

All classrooms are acoustically treated and each has no more than 25 children per fully qualified kindergarten teacher and a

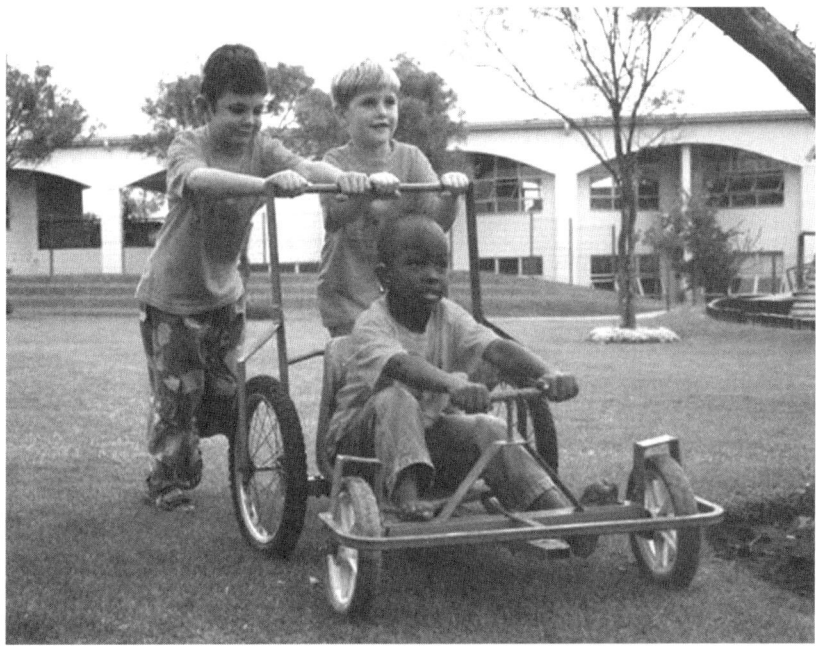

Figure 6–3. Social skills develop as children play together in a South African program..

learning support assistant. FM systems are used in all classrooms. Attached to each class is a small room that can be used for small group work or for individual conversation. Children with hearing loss spend one more hour in the program each day than those with normal hearing. This allows for each hearing-impaired child to have three different linguistic experiences per day:

- Full participation in all language group work alongside their classmates with normal hearing
- Additional work in small groups comprised only of hearing-impaired children; work is based on the linguistic level of the child
- An individual conversation.

In addition, parents have regular guidance sessions as often as is needed.

The Primary School Stage

Audiological Management

When compulsory school age is reached, prior to the placement of children with a hearing loss in a mainstream primary school, personnel in mainstream schools need special training. On the audiologic side, the regular school staff needs to understand:

- the importance of daylong listening
- the basic features of the hearing aids and cochlear implants as well as how to check their efficiency at the start of each school day
- how to create the best possible listening environment—avoiding all unnecessary background noise (e.g., air conditioners, fans, etc.)
- the effective use of the FM systems
- the importance of training the child to alert someone if the hearing aid/system is not working properly
- whom to contact if there is a problem with the hearing instruments. Loaner hearing aids/cochlear implant processors should be available for times when equipment needs to be sent off for repair. It is very disturbing for a pupil with hearing loss to be without amplification even for a day.

When there is a child with hearing loss in a class, the staff needs to be aware that they should:

- keep unwanted classroom noise to a minimum
- always speak in the same way to the child with a hearing loss as to the class as a whole (no exaggerated mouth movements or slower rate of utterance)
- ensure that the child sits where the teacher's face can be seen
- avoid walking up and down a center passage when giving important information because the hearing-impaired child cannot see the teacher's normal facial expressions
- expect the same standard of behavior from the child as from those with normal hearing
- expect the child to take part in group or class discussions

- avoid habits like emphasizing a point by tapping on the board (this is disturbing when heard through a hearing aid)
- encourage the child to speak up when he or she does not understand
- understand the possibility that the child will be at a more limited linguistic level than at least some of the other children
- check how much the child is understanding the general classwork on a regular basis

On this subject it is interesting to read an article by a parent, Gordon-Langbein (2001), summarizing many of the most important areas.

Linguistic Development

There are many different patterns of inclusion currently developing worldwide. The Canossian School in Singapore realized the advantages of inclusive education early on. A site on the same campus as an established primary school was chosen as the relocation point for the CSHI School (now CSH). An Eduplex has developed here. This includes:

- a regular kindergarten
- a mainstream primary school
- the Canossian school catering to and supporting children with a hearing loss
- a Children's Home
- a Convent.

This primary school lacks physical space, but uses this to its advantage, having two sessions per day (for example, grades 2, 4, and 6 in the morning and grades 1, 3, and 5 in the afternoon). It has therefore been possible to implement a unique and very efficient model of inclusion whose main features are:

- full inclusion in the mainstream school for either the whole morning or whole afternoon session
- an additional two hours of support work for hearing-impaired children in the neighboring CSH building, either before or after the the mainstream school session. This

allows for tutorial work on the primary school curriculum and continuing general linguistic development
- close relationship between the class teacher in the mainstream setting and the CSH support teacher
- FM system for each included child
- on-site audiologic management of each child.
- on-site hearing aid maintenance
- regular training sessions for the mainstream school staff

The system implemented for Pretoria Eduplex preschool in South Africa is merging with the primary school very successfully. At the primary school level, the support offered is increased to 1½ hours daily. The staff is aware of the need for the three types of daily linguistic experience, and they realize that hearing-impaired children, in addition to learning the curriculum's subjects, must generally be led to a more accurate and mature level of linguistic competence. This is best done through regular sessions of individual conversation in which the specific linguistic needs of each child can be detected and addressed. The type of support offered needs to be examined critically.

It is not always easy to persuade those offering support to hearing-impaired children in other countries to spend time on general language development. It is easy to locate gaps in their knowledge related to the subjects of the curriculum and, in many cases, almost all the available support time is used filling these gaps.

Like the South African program the Ecuadorian program is addressing this issue well and demonstrating that, the link between general linguistic capability and progress in the academic program becomes obvious when proper time is allocated.

All over the world, children with hearing loss attend regular school with varying degrees of support. Observation shows that the degree to which this support meets the individual needs of the child determines, to a large extent, the program's success. In some cases, where education authorities have well-planned support services, hearing-impaired children really are "included" and are doing very well. In others, however, many children are struggling with insufficient support and the term "included" cannot be applied in such situations.

For some programs, too much dependence on parents can be a worrisome feature. "Homework" sent home with the child often takes many hours to complete each night and each weekend. Anxious to keep the child in the included setting, parents struggle to cope, but at the expense of their ability to serve the needs of the whole family. One parent recently summed this up when she said,

> Our family life has suffered since she (a girl with severe hearing loss) went into primary school. If we don't sit with her with the homework, she just can't cope in class, because she does not seem to learn much by herself there. We no longer have time to do fun things and our two other children are beginning to resent this.

Homework should keep the parents aware of what is being covered in class and provide the child with an opportunity to consolidate it as the parents take, perhaps, a different angle on the subject. It should not, however, be laborious for parents to teach the child something new nor should they struggle with something that was not understood in class. Reducing the amount of set homework is not the solution. What matters is that the teacher understands what is within the capability of the child and assigns homework at an attainable level.

It is sad to find that financial restraints have caused some education authorities to opt for "inclusion" in order to avoid the fees that come with special schools. Inclusion should not be considered a cheap option. If adequate support is to be provided for all who need to be included, the expense will be little, if any, less than fees for residential educational placement. As more and more children continue to be included, it is hoped that authorities will gradually accept responsibility for providing the necessary degree of support and conditions for children in included situations will improve.

Professionals who know the special needs of a particular child with a hearing loss have a responsibility to be critical of each opportunity to be offered for inclusion. It is wiser to delay inclusion in countries where there are large numbers of children in noisy classrooms and poorly trained teachers, FM equipment is not available, and no preliminary support or preparation has been offered to the mainstream school under consideration. Seeing the success of some well-run inclusion programs, it is understandable to want to see others develop quickly, but caution must be exercised. Over the 20 years during which the author has been involved in international work, it has often been necessary to insist on thorough preparation of a few pilot projects rather than place hearing-impaired children in situations where it would not be possible for them to cope successfully.

Another area of concern is when a preschool facility is coping well with hearing-impaired children and promises parents that the natural next step for their child will be a regular mainstream school. This promise should be made only if a suitable primary school can be identified where the necessary support is available to ensure the child's special needs are met. Observation in several countries shows that, if this is not done, false hopes may be raised. These can lead to feelings of disappointment and failure on the part of both parent and child. This situation is further complicated by the fact that, for the first year or two of primary school, all may appear to be going well, but the child's basic difficulties may not be identified. In such cases, as curriculum demands increase in the later grades, the hearing-impaired child may be unable to cope. Adequate support and thorough ongoing assessment are absolute essentials.

The Secondary School Stage

Audiological Management

In Britain, it is common practice to have a promoted post for a "special needs coordinator" of a secondary school. It is important for this staff member to develop a good rapport with hearing-impaired students. Whether or not an official post of this kind exists in an inclusionary school, it is important for pupils with special needs to know which staff member they may go to when problems arise.

Students should be trained to take more responsibility for their own needs; for example they should be responsible for checking the condition of their hearing aids as much as possible. By secondary school age, pupils can evaluate their own hearing aids, and it is important to listen to their views. A wide choice of hearing aids is available today and the support service should be aware of the latest models and be prepared to change hearing aids if better responses are obtained from a newer model.

Although the size of FM equipment has now been overcome, pupils in their teens are often self-conscious about having to hand the transmitter of an FM system from teacher to teacher. Each staff member who deals with the hearing-impaired pupil needs to be aware of the value of using an FM system and insist on its use.

Linguistic Development

Life can become more difficult for hearing-impaired students at the secondary school level because, in any one day, they may be taught by five or six different teachers across a range of subjects. Technical language may become much more involved at an age in the pupil's life when he or she is sensitive about asking for help. No single support teacher can adequately deal with the content of the whole secondary school curriculum. This means that support for the pupil must be given by special subject teachers rather than by specialists in deaf education. It is important for these subject teachers to receive training in the probable linguistic problems of the hearing-impaired and general classroom practices that will allow a hearing-impaired child to have full access to the curriculum.

In Singapore, one secondary school has enrolled several pupils with hearing loss. The principal has been very faithful in asking for regular workshops to ensure that any new members of staff are introduced to the probable difficulties caused by the presence of hearing loss. Timetables have been arranged so that the subject teachers with hearing-impaired pupils in their classes have time set aside in which they are free to offer support to these pupils in a small group or on an individual basis. This has been a most satisfactory approach.

In England, DELTA (2003) has produced valuable videotaped evidence of interviews of a group of hearing-impaired students who left school at age 16 or older. All these young people were educated in inclusive situations in five different English counties. Their academic results matched the level of their normally hearing peers and their reading levels were age-appropriate, some even ahead of their chronological ages. On the videotape, they speak for themselves about their experiences. On this tape, there are examples of the type of inclusion they enjoyed, because today's preschool and primary school children are observed in their present inclusive situations.

Other Considerations

Reverse Integration

In a few countries where problems have arisen when hearing-impaired children were accepted in regular schools, non-hearing-impaired children with normal hearing have been invited to attend a special school for children with a hearing loss. The aim was twofold:

- to provide the with normal hearing children with a more supportive learning environment than is available in large mainstream classes
- to surround the hearing-impaired children with as much normal, natural language as possible.

In some cases this has worked well. In others there have been some serious concerns:

- The with normal hearing children put forward for such a scheme may be those with language-learning problems or those with low innate ability. This increases the pressure on staff dealing with the linguistic problems of hearing-impaired children.
- The with normal hearing children may be unhappy about the small numbers in a special school and may miss the opportunities for competitive sport, and so forth.
- Due to their size, special schools are not always able to offer as wide a curriculum as the regular school.

Specialization in Inclusion

The worldwide movement toward inclusion on the whole, recommends that neighborhood mainstream schools should accept all children in their area despite their special needs. This may work well in a large school where there are several classes at each level but the implications of such a philosophy must be fully understood. If there are to be several children with different problems in one class:

- It would be difficult for any one teacher to acquire the necessary skills to deal in depth with a variety of handicaps in a single class and to meet each child's individual needs efficiently.
- Pressure placed on the teacher by the inclusion of several children with very different special needs would make it difficult to maintain a high enough standard to ensure that all children in the class reach their full potential.
- It would be extremely complex to organize enough support to meet each child's special needs efficiently.

With the above concerns in mind, the Eduplex in Pretoria, South Africa was planned to concentrate on the inclusion of hearing-impaired children only. This realistic practice ensures that high standards can be maintained for all the children. Staff training was needed in only one specialized area, which made in-depth training possible across the range of areas connected with deafness. This ensures the needs of the children with a hearing loss are being met efficiently.

The movement toward worldwide inclusion highlights the need for cooperation among all concerned. Expectations of everyone involved are being raised. Parents, specialists, mainstream teachers, and those with the power to implement inclusion need to come together to identify the strengths and weaknesses of each program. Undoubtedly, it will take time for the segregated pattern of special education still practiced in many places today to diminish and be replaced by a truly inclusive model.

Only with careful planning, professional training, and the provision of necessary resources in personnel and equipment can the special needs of children with hearing impairment be adequately met in educational settings allowing full access to the curriculum. Smith (2002) sums up the situation when he notes that it is necessary for there to be a shift of focus from the mere availability of service to the quality of education that children with special needs receive in inclusive situations.

CHAPTER 7

The Way Forward

> *"Under normal circumstances, spoken language is the key to the full realization of human potential."*
>
> **(Boothroyd, 2000)**

The motivation for this book came from over 50 years of practice in the education of hearing-impaired children around the world. Its findings have been based on five kinds of experience:

- A solid foundation of experience with normally hearing children in the early stages of language development and early education
- Hands-on work with children suffering from all degrees of deafness
- Many years guiding parents and caregivers of children with a hearing loss in their overall management of the child
- Training teachers and students engaged in or preparing for work with hearing-impaired children. This includes planning new degree and diploma courses in the Natural Auditory Oral approach
- Observation of and involvement in programs worldwide, in which professionals are committed to moving forward and taking advantage of all that is available today.

The half-century and more that this text covers has been exciting due to advances in audiology, hearing aid technology, medical science, and psycholinguistics. Through tracing progress due to these new opportunities, this book has illustrated how what is now available can provide a quality of life for today's children with a hearing loss that was previously only a dream. The realization that today's children with severe and profound hearing losses can hear and can therefore follow the normal language learning pattern of a child with normal hearing has revolutionized practice in many areas.

Unfortunately these opportunities are not yet available for all hearing-impaired children in developed or developing countries. If things are to change in the future it is necessary to analyze the reasons why:

- Some reasons are basic and depend merely on the lack of resources in underdeveloped areas. The solution to these problems is obvious. There is a responsibility for those in developed countries to share experiences, offer training, and help in the provision of resources that will make necessary training and equipment available.
- In other areas, the problem is a political one whose roots lie deep in the history of education for deaf children. Those who desire to preserve "Deaf culture," after recognizing the failure of "Total Communication" programs, have introduced what they call "Bilingualism." This places little or no emphasis on the use of the child's residual hearing at the language-learning stage and does not take advantage of what is available today. Lane and Bahan (1998) argued against cochlear implants when, talking about the 60,000 children who receive special services for the hearing impaired in the United States of America, they say, "With a perfect implant available, most would be candidates for the surgery. Thus the population of the Deaf World in the United States would decline drastically . . . This must be a matter of great ethical concern."
- In therapy-dominated early intervention programs, the emphasis is on childen being "taught" to listen and to speak while parents watch. The emphasis in an observational approach should be on offering advice to parents based on observation of their particular needs and those of their child. Parents should not be turned into teachers, but

rather should be educated on how to provide an environment in which the children "learn" to listen and speak. If not, when parents and children do not make the expected progress in the more formal programs, they often drop out and the children are considered unsuitable for "oral education."

The author observed a very anxious parent interacting with her three-year-old daughter. "We have to do prepositions," she said, "but I can't get her to say, 'between.'" The mother then held up a photograph and said, "She has to be able to say, 'I am standing between my mother and my brother' and she can't do it. I'm not going back there." Fifteen percent of the hearing-impaired children in one Natural Auditory Oral program in which the author is working have transferred from therapy-dominated programs. They are developing well in the more natural situation.

Over the years, the author has found that low expectations of professionals are based on lack of exposure to all that is possible today. This is a major cause for acceptance of the status quo and the maintenance of low standards.

All of this can change. Many professionals and parents today have been privileged to work with children having severe and profound hearing loss. These children's language has developed to a level that allowed fulfillment of their academic potential as well as linguistic independence for life.

At the beginning of the 21st century there is a developing awareness of the need to publicize what is possible and what has been happening in various independent programs all over the world. In some cases this has been going on for many years.

The DELTA literature provides examples of pioneers for the future, capable of demonstrating what is possible. However, earlier than the DELTA material, living proof, offered in the form of five videotapes of linguistically capable young people from the former Birkdale School for the Hearing Impaired in England, (Clark, 1984) caused the Canossian School in Singapore during the 1980s to drop Total Communication entirely and adopt the Natural Auditory Oral approach (see Chapter 6). So successful was this that it is now a wholly auditory oral program, more than 70% of whose pupils are fully included in mainstream schools. Nor are they satisfied with that. Plans are already underway to move to a program for inclusion of all pupils. Its first stage has begun in 2006.

Aware of the need to keep abreast of modern developments, an approach was made to Nan Yang University in Singapore and an Advanced Diploma Course on the Natural Auditory Oral approach is now running as a two-year part-time course.

Others have been similarly influenced by an introduction to today's possibilities and have been motivated to implement change or begin completely new programs. These include:

- The Natural Auditory Oral program in Eskisehir, in Anadolu University, Turkey where, in addition to the children's program, there is now a four-year degree course for teachers of the hearing impaired based on the Natural Auditory Oral approach.
- Nippon Rowa Gakko (Japan's Oral School) in Tokyo
- A small program on the tiny Mauritian island of Rodrigues
- The three programs operating on the basic principles of the Natural Auditory Oral approach in Ecuador
- Elsewhere the emphasis has changed from a traditional to a more natural approach in several programs, for example, in Saskatchewan (Canada) and in some German and Hungarian programs.

One of the most forward-looking programs today, the result of very careful planning, has much to teach us as we look to the future. It is the Eduplex in Pretoria, South Africa—the brainchild of one South African businessman. He was passionate about implementing change to improve conditions for children who have hearing loss. From the start he decided to confine any inclusion program to children whose special needs arose from one handicap only—hearing impairment. This program can serve as a model for the way forward because:

- Aware of today's possibilities, old standards were no longer acceptable and there was real motivation to change.
- The support of the neighboring Ear Institute ensures very efficient testing of hearing as well as the fitting of appropriate hearing aids and their maintenance, plus supplying four full-time audiologists to the Eduplex program.
- Realizing the need to share the vision with professionals who could implement the necessary changes, training courses in the new approach were organized and are still ongoing.

- Professionals motivated to make a change were identified.
- Financial resources were sought and were initially, generously provided by Swiss donors.
- Keeping abreast of the worldwide movement toward inclusion, a mainstream educational program was established with the aim of including 20% children with a hearing loss.
- The larger than normal proportion of hearing-impaired children removes the feeling of isolation reported by many who have been the only hearing-impaired child in the whole school.
- When 20% of the class has a hearing loss, teachers cannot ignore the need to plan work linguistically so as to include their needs.
- A strong parent guidance program forms the basis of a planned inclusion program for the hearing-impaired children and it continues through the primary school years. It is compulsory for parents of children who have hearing loss to attend parent guidance programs.
- The gardens surrounding the buildings were planned to provide opportunities for language extension as children become involved in activities around the bird yard, the pond, and so forth (see Figure 7–1).

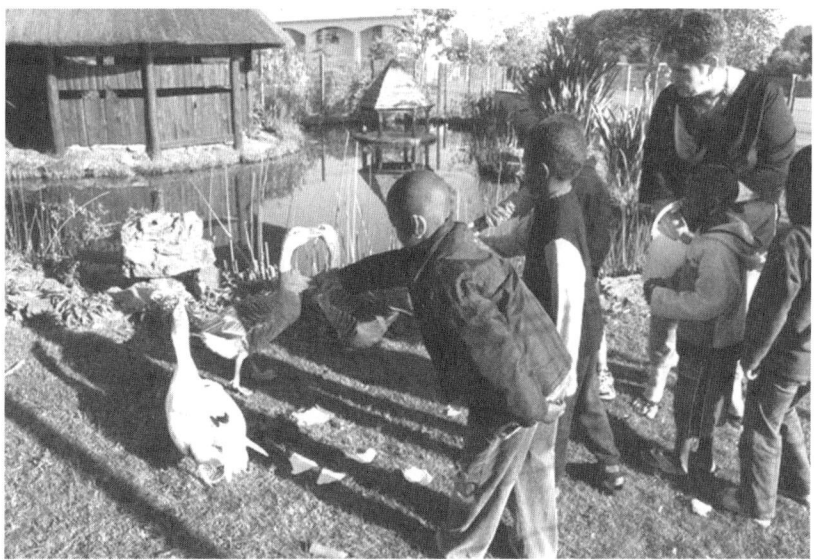

Figure 7–1. Responsibility of caring for animals necessitates interaction.

- Children with hearing loss take full part in all activities. Sports offers many informal situations for social development (see Figure 7–2).
- A group teaching approach meets a range of needs for children in a class and ensures that children learn to work independently (see Figure 7–3).
- The children with hearing losses spend 1½ hours longer in school each day to allow time for the necessary support provided in small groups or individual time with the teacher. This ensures they will not be withdrawn from class during normal school hours.
- The support offered to the children with a hearing loss is given by their own teachers who know exactly the individual needs of each child.
- Grants were sought for children from economically poor homes to ensure attendance.

Time was taken at the planning stage to list the ways in which the building, the environment, and the educational approach should be adapted to the needs of children with a hearing loss, including:

- Acoustic treatment of all classrooms to allow the best possible listening conditions. Although this was planned specifically for

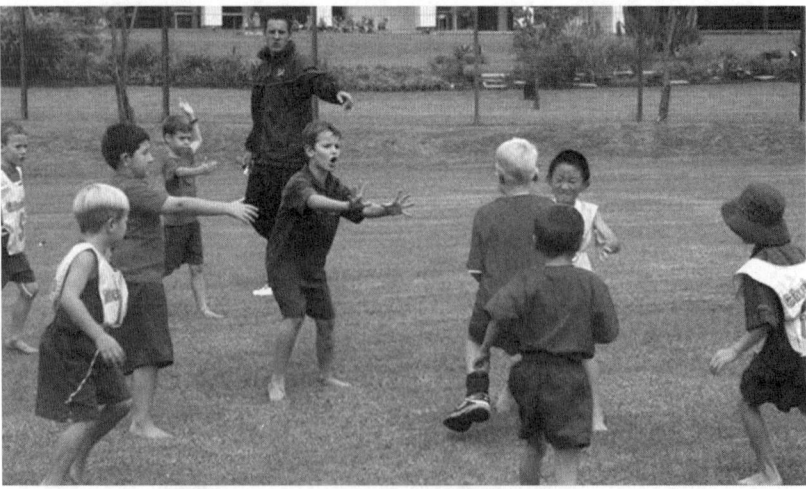

Figure 7–2. Learning to be part of a team in sports activities

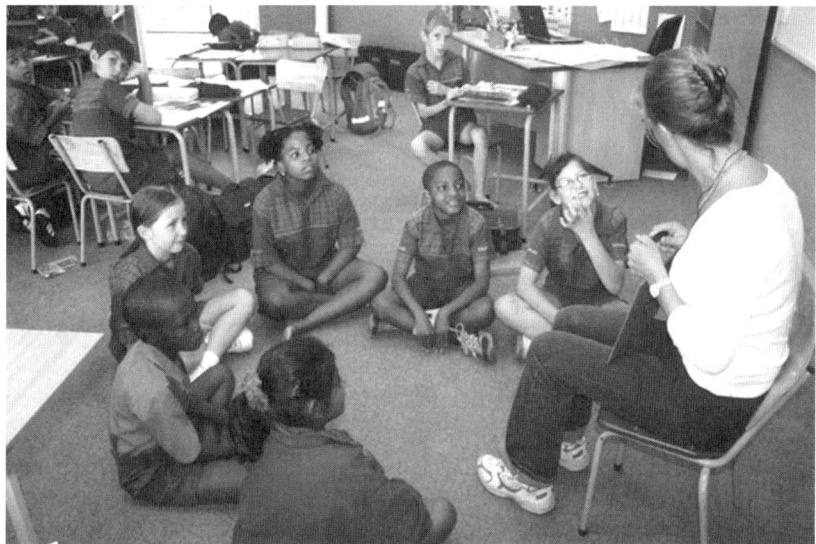

Figure 7–3. *Group work offers support and ensures development of independent work habits.*

the hearing-impaired children with normal hearing children benefit tremendously from the good acoustic environment.

■ Small rooms, adjacent to each classroom, in which individual conversations and small-group work, are geared specifically to the linguistic needs of the hearing-impaired students.

■ A staff/pupil ratio of teachers and classroom assistants allows the teacher to carry out small group work and individual conversation work with the hearing-impaired children while simultaneously ensuring that the children with normal hearing are adequately stimulated and supervised (25 children per class with a teacher and classroom assistant).

■ A specially planned, linguistically motivating environment both indoors and out. This includes various features in the gardens that provide a basis for discussion and stimulate interaction.

■ In addition to the regular educational staff, four audiologists/ speech therapists manage the parent guidance program, attend to the specific audiologic and linguistic needs of the children with a hearing loss, and provide ongoing training for staff of both the preschool and primary school.

- A training facility was also established which allows for many courses of different levels to be provided for:
  - Those wishing to hear of the approach and see its application (audiologists, speech and language therapists, medical personnel, and students).
  - Those seriously considering implementing change in South Africa and other countries.
  - Those interested in the general implementation of inclusion, apart from those directly connected with hearing-impaired children.

The author considers it a privilege to be associated with this program, and its results have reinforced her conviction that, even in very difficult circumstances, conditions for today's hearing-impaired children can be revolutionized. No two programs will be identical but, where professionals are fired with the vision to be agents of change and are given the necessary training in the practical application of the changes required, dreams really can become realities.

Bibliography

Abberton, E., et al. (1987) Speech pattern acquisition in profoundly hearing impaired children. *Proceedings of the XIth International Congress of Phonetic Sciences*, Tallinn, Estonia, USSR.

Archbold, S. (2005). Cochlear implants. In W. McCracken & S. Laoide-Kemp (Eds.), *Audiology in education.* London: Whurr.

Bamford, J., & McSporran, E. (1993). Early detection and diagnosis of hearing impairment: A United Kingdom perspective. *Volta Review*, 95(5).

Batliner G, (2004), *Horgeschadigte Kinder Spielerisch Forde.* Munich: Ernst Reinhardt Verlag.

Beebe, H. (1953). *A guide to help the severely hard of hearing child.* Basel/New York: Karger.

Bloom, P. (2000). *How children learn the meaning of words.* Cambridge MA: MIT Press.

Boothroyd, A. (2000). Management of hearing loss in children: No simple solutions. In R. C. Seewald (Ed.), *A sound foundation through early amplification* (pp. 1–12). Zurich, Switzerland: Phonak AG.

Brackett, D., & Pollack, D, (1986). Auditory learning. *Volta Review*, 85(5).

Brown, M. (2002). Systemic, family, parent and child factors associated with the rate of spoken language development in young children with profound hearing loss. In *Developing the listening ear.* Haverhill, Suffolk: DELTA

Brown, P. M., & Carey-Sargent, C. (2001). Assessing early spoken language interaction between a hearing mother and an infant with a profound hearing loss. *Deafness and Education International*, 3(2), 49–61.

Bruner, J. (1983). *Child's talk.* Oxford: Oxford University Press.

Carey-Sargeant, C. L., & Brown, P. M. (2003). Pausing during interactions between deaf toddlers and their hearing mothers. *Deafness and Education International*, 5(1), 39–58.

Carpenter B., Ashdown R., & Bovair, K. (1996). *Enabling access: Effective teaching and learning for students with learning difficulties.* London: David Fulton.

Chute, P. M., & Nevins, M. E. (2006). *School professionals working with children with cochlear implants.* San Diego, CA: Plural Publishing.

Clark, M. (1985-6). *Developing the spoken language skills of hearing impaired children* [series of five one-hour videotapes with written commentaries]. Manchester, UK: MUTV Manchester University.

Clark, M. (1989). *Language through living.* London: Hodder and Stoughton.

Clark, M. (1998). Overview of educational provision for hearing impaired children: From 1950 to the present. *Seminars in Hearing, 18*(3).

Clark, M. (2002). Listening around the world in proceedings of the Delta Conference. *Developing the listening ear.* Haverhill, Suffolk: DELTA.

Clark, M., & Tan, A. (2004). Learners with hearing loss. In L. Lim & M. Quah (Eds.), *Educating learners with diverse abilities* (chap. 12). Singapore: McGraw-Hill.

Clark, M., & Tufekcioglu, U. (1994). Developing a comprehensive service for the hearing impaired in Turkey. *Journal of the British Association of Teachers of the Deaf, 18*(3), 82–85.

Cole, E. B. (1992). *Listening and talking.* Washington, DC: A.G. Bell.

Compton, M., V., Niemeyer, J. A., & Michael, S. (2003). Auditory /oral birth-kindergarten teacher preparation: A research based model. *Volta Review, 104*(2), 93–106.

Crystal, D. (1997). *The Cambridge encyclopedia of language* (2nd ed.). Cambridge: Cambridge University Press.

Corcoran, J. A., et al. (2000). Stories of parents of children with hearing loss. In R. Seewald (Ed.), *A sound foundation through early amplification.* Zurich, Switzerland: Phonak AG.

DELTA. (1999). *Deaf children talking: The parents' guide to the Natural Aural Approach.* Haverhill, Suffolk, UK: DELTA.

DELTA. (2003). *Sound futures* [Videotape with written commentary]. Haverhill, Suffolk, UK: DELTA.

Dillier, N. (2005). Combining cochlear implants and hearing instruments. In R. C. Seewald & J. M. Bamford (Eds.), *A sound foundation through early amplification* (pp. 163–172). Zurich, Switzerland: Phonak AG.

Duncan, J. (1999). Conversational skills of children with hearing loss and children with normal; hearing in an integrated setting. *Volta Review, 101*(4), 193–211.

Ewing, I. R., & Ewing, A. W. G. (1954). *Speech and the deaf child.* Manchester, UK: Manchester University Press.

Fry, D., & Whetnall, E. (1954) The auditory approach in the training of deaf children. *Lancet, 266*, 583–587.

Geers A., Moog, J., & Schick, B. (1984) Acquisition of spoken and signed English by profoundly deaf children. *Journal of Speech and Hearing Disorders, 49*, 378-388.

Gordon-Langbein, A. (2001, October). 9 things to know about listening and learning in today's classrooms. *Volta Voices*, pp. 23-27.

Hall, J. (2001). *Paediatric hearing assessment.* Paper presented at the Phonak Paediatric Conference, Pretoria, South Africa.

Hanko, G. (1995). *Special needs in ordinary classrooms, from staff support to staff development.* London: David Fulton.

Harrison, M., & Roush, J. (2001). Information for families of young deaf and hard of hearing children. In R. Seewald & J. Gravel (Eds.), *Proceedings of the Second International Conference: A sound foundation through early amplification* (pp. 233-249). Zurich, Switzerland: Phonak AG.

Holmans, A. (2005, May). Early years support. *BATOD Magazine*, p. 9.

Holt, J. (1970). *How children learn* (pp. 57-58). Harmondsworth, UK: Penguin Books.

Kretschmer, R., & Kretschmer, L. (1978). *Language development and interaction with the hearing impaired.* Baltimore: University Park Press.

Lane, H., & Bahan, B. (1998). Ethics of cochlear implantation in young children: A review and reply from a Deaf World perspective. *Otolaryngology-Head and Neck Surgery, 119(4)*, 297-313.

Lieven, E. V. M. (1984. Interactional styles and children's language learning. *Topics in Language Disorders, 4(4)*, 15-23.

Lim, L., & Tam, J. (2004). Learning and diversity. In L. Lim & M. M. Quah (Eds.), *Educating learners with diverse abilities* (pp.1-28). Singapore: McGraw-Education.

Lock, A. (1980). *The guided reinvention of language.* London: Academic Press.

Lowe, A. (1990, July). *The history of auditory education seen from the European point of view.* Presentation at Alexander Graham Bell Association Convention, Washington, DC.

Lynas, W. (1994). *Communication options in the education of deaf children.* London: Whurr.

Lynas, W., Huntington, A., & Tucker, I. (1988) *A critical examination of different approaches to communication in the education of deaf children.* Manchester, UK: The Ewing Foundation.

Markides, A. (1988). Speech intelligibility: Auditory oral approach versus total communication. *Journal of the British Association of Teachers of the Deaf, 12(6)*, 136-141.

McCracken, W., et al. (2005). The impact of NHSP on educational services in England. *Deafness and Education International, 7(4)*, 179-184.

McAnally, P., Rose, S., & Quigley, S. (1987*). Language learning practices with deaf children.* Boston: College-Hill Press.

Mittler, P. (2000). *Working towards inclusive education: Social contexts.* London: David Fulton.

Morrison, E. F., Rimm-Kauffman, S., & Pianta, R. C. (2003). A longitudinal study of mother child interactions at school entry and social and academic outcomes in middle school. *Journal of School Psychology, 41*(3), 185–200.

Most, T. (2004). The effects of degree and types of hearing loss on children's performance in class. *Deafness and Education International, 6*(3), 154–166.

Nevins, M., & Chute, P. (2006*). Children with cochlear implants in an educational setting.* San Diego, CA: Plural Publishing.

Northern, J. L., & Downs M. P. (1991). *Hearing in children* (4th ed.). Baltimore: Williams & Wilkins.

Papousek, H., & Papousek, M. (1992). Beyond emotional bonding: The role of preverbal communication in mental growth and health. *Infant Mental Health Journal, 13*(1), 43–53.

Paul, P. (1988). American sign language and English: A bilingual minority language immersion programme. *Conference of American Instructors of the Deaf, News 'N' Notes.* Washington, DC: American Instructors of the Deaf.

Paul, P., & Quigley, S. (1994). *Language and deafness.* San Diego, CA: Singular Publishing Group.

Pinker, S. (1994). *The language instinct.* New York: HarperCollins.

Pollack, D. (1985). *Educational audiology for the limited-hearing infant and preschooler* (2nd ed.). Springfield, IL: Charles C. Thomas.

Pritchard, D. G. (1963). *Education and the handicapped.* London: Routledge and Kegan Paul.

Proctor, R., Niemeyer, J. A., & Compton, M. V. (2005). Training needs of early intervention workers with infants and toddlers who are deaf or hard of hearing. *Volta Review, 105*(2), 113–128.

Quigley, S., & Kretschmer, R. E. (1982). *The education of deaf children.* London: Edward Arnold.

Robertson, L., & Flexer, C. (2000). *Literacy learning for children who are deaf or hard of hearing.* Washington, DC: Alexander Graham Bell Association for the Deaf.

Ross, M. (1986). A perspective on amplification: Then and now. In D. M. Luterman (Ed.), *Deafness in perspective.* San Diego, CA: College-Hill Press.

Smith, D. (2002). *Introduction to special education* (4th ed.). Needham Heights, MA: Allyn & Bacon.

Snow, C. E. (1977). The development of conversation between mothers and babies. *Journal of Child Language*, *4*, 1-22.

Stern, D. N., Spieker, S., Barnett, R. K., & McKain, K. (1983). The prosody of maternal speech: Infant age and context related changes. *Journal of Child Language*, *10*, 1-15.

Stokes, J. (Ed.). (1999). *Hearing impaired infants—Support in the first 18 months*. London: Whurr.

Strauss, S. (2006). *Early hearing intervention and support services provided to the paediatric population by South African audiologists* (pp. 200-201). Unpublished thesis, Department of Communication Pathology, University of Pretoria.

Sugarman, S. (1983). Empirical versus logical issues in the transition from prelinguistic to linguistic communication. In R. M. Golinkoff (Ed.), *The transition from paralinguistic to linguistic communication*. Hillsdale NJ: Lawrence Erlbaum.

Tabors, P. O. (1997). *One child, two languages: A guide for preschool educators of children learning English as a second language*. Baltimore: Paul H. Brookes.

Tait, M. (1986). Using singing to facilitate linguistic development in hearing impaired pre-schoolers. *Journal of the British Association of Teachers of the Deaf*, *10*(4).

Tassoni, P., & Hucker, K. (2000). *Planning play and the early years*. Oxford: Heinemann Educational Publishers.

van Uden, A. (1977). *A world of language for deaf children* (3rd ed.). Amsterdam: Swets & Zeitlinger.Tough, J. (1977). *The development of meaning*. London: Allen and Unwin.

Vihman, M. M. (1996). *Phonological development: The origins of language in the child*. Oxford: Blackwell.

Wells, G. (1979). Variation in child language. In P. Fletcher & M. Garman (Eds.), *Language acquisition*. Cambridge: Cambridge University Press.

Wells, G. (1986). *The meaning makers*. London: Hodder and Stoughton.

Whetnall, E., & Fry, D. (1964). *The deaf child*. London: Heinemann

Wood, D., Wood, H., Griffiths, A., & Howarth, I. (1986) *Teaching and talking with deaf children*. Chichester, UK: John Wiley and Sons.

Yoshinago-Itano, C. (2001). *Universal newborn hearing screening*. Paper presented at the Phonak Paediatric Conference, Pretoria, South Africa.

APPENDIX A

Overview of Developments from Mid-20th Century Onward[*]

To understand the present day situation in the education of children with a hearing loss, it is necessary to consider it in light of the major developments in the field. It must be realized that many of today's adult deaf who were educated in so-called "oral schools" left school unable to either speak or sign well. They are justifiably anxious that children with hearing impairment today should have better treatment and better opportunities than they had and many are demanding a say in the educational provision made for the hearing impaired. What is not clearly understood is the difference that advances in the field of medicine, technology, audiology, and psycholinguistics have made to the opportunities available to children with a hearing loss in the 21st century. Today's natural auditory oral programs, which have the use of hearing as their base line, are as different from the old "oral" programs as these were from the signing programs that preceded them.

---

[*]Updated and adapted with permission from Clark, M. "Overview of educational provision for hearing-impaired children: From 1950 to the present," *Seminars in Hearing, 18*(3). Copyright 1998 Thieme.

Around the 1950s

The author writes from firsthand experience of the time from 1954 onward in England, but the situation in many other European countries and in the United States at that time was similar, although not identical. In the period immediately after World War II, there were only two alternatives for the educational placement of a child who was hearing impaired. One was placement in a Special School for the Deaf (very often a residential special school) and the other was placement in the child's regular neighborhood school without any form of support to cater for special educational needs, unless parents were in a position to provide that privately.

Toward the end of the 1940s another alternative became available in England. Schools for the Partially Hearing began to open. The first of these opened in 1948 in Birkdale, Southport and three others followed shortly after. This option came about, in no small measure, due to the development of the pure tone audiometer and the ability to measure the degree of hearing loss. The awareness that some children who had a hearing loss could hear something of speech was a significant development and was the first step toward the raising of expectations. From the start, the whole approach in these schools in Britain was one that followed as closely as possible that of the regular school. The classification of children at that time was that those with hearing losses up to 60 dB were considered to be partially hearing and all born with hearing losses over 60 dB were considered to be deaf.

The opening of Partially Hearing Schools had an immediate effect on the population of Schools for the Deaf. Until that time there had been children in Schools for the Deaf who had hearing losses of 60 dB and less. For the most part, those were the children who had developed some fluency and intelligibility of spoken language and who gave the impression that all was well within the schools. When this group of children left, the situation was very different. The low levels of communicative competence of the majority of children within the Schools for the Deaf became apparent.

Educationally, in Schools for the Deaf, in the postwar period up to 1957 things went on much as they had for decades before because modern hearing aids had not become freely available and the old valve hearing aids were cumbersome and were really not practical for constant use by very young children. There was little knowledge about the residual hearing of the children placed there (e.g., the author entered a traditional school for the deaf in Scotland in 1955 and had no access to any audiological data concerning the children in the class for whom she was responsible.) It is very important to know what *did* happen in those years before the availability of modern hearing aids, because practices adopted then lingered on throughout much of the period that followed and many of these practices are detrimental to the development of spoken language. Some still exist today in areas where it is difficult for professionals to keep abreast of modern techniques.

Most of the schools claimed to run "oral" programs, but few, if any, saw hearing aids as essential to the process of the development of spoken language to a level that would prepare the students for life in hearing society. Although available in some situations, the old valve hearing aids were not worn all day long and children were certainly not "hearing aid dependent." In fact, the programs were at best "oral" in the classrooms only (Kretschmer & Kretschmer, 1978.) The level and type of language that the children developed there was insufficient for living and, in most situations outside of classrooms, the children communicated with each other by using signs.

It was reasoned that deaf children could not hear and this was true because, without hearing aids, most of the children in the schools could not hear. The logical conclusion was, therefore, to substitute "eyes for ears." This led to the adoption of all sorts of abnormal practices in the attempt to bring children to the use of spoken language. If children could not hear, it was reasoned, they must receive language through the eyes and this was taken to mean through *lipreading.* The children's attention had to be drawn to the lips and this was constantly done by exhorting the children to *"watch,"* often with a visual clue from the teacher as she or he pointed to the lips. From this, developed the habit of *exaggerating lip movements* in an attempt to make lipreading easier. This, in fact, distorted normal patterns of speech, and often broke up the features of rhythm and intonation that are so important to intelligibility. A further measure taken to make lipreading easier was *to select words that were easy to lipread* and make lists of vocabulary that consisted of such words, usually grouping these around a certain topic (e.g., apple, banana, plum, orange, etc.). These were then taught to children *as single words* and lots of lipreading exercises were given. Almost all the words used in the early stages were very concrete and objects associated with these *were held up to the lips* so that the object could be associated with the lipread pattern. Through these practices children accepted that the "way in" to language was through the eyes and little was done to stimulate residual hearing.

The whole thinking about language learning was very different from our concept of that area today. It was assumed that one must begin with single words and then take measures to ensure that sentence patterns were taught. All the language introduced was adult imposed and little thought was given to empowering children to give them the chance to become independent language learners and so to acquire the language that they needed to express their thoughts and feelings. After a small vocabulary of nouns had been built up, teachers would start to *teach short phrases* (e.g., linking an object and its color, for example, a yellow banana, a red apple, etc.). In time this would be *developed into short sentences, but these were for the most part artificial* (e.g., The apple is red. The banana is yellow). Such sentences were taught to the child who was expected to produce them when asked. This language was sterile and had no emotive content.

The awareness of the difficulty of lipreading fleeting patterns on the lips led to the practice of introducing the written form of the words and sentences early, in the hope that the children would develop spoken language from the written word—another visual way in.

Without hearing aids, children with significant hearing losses could learn to lipread some of these words, but might try to copy them without the use of voice (i.e., by mere lip movements). Even when they did vocalize, their attempts to imitate speech and their voice quality were, for the most part, very poor. As a result, the practice of "teaching speech" from a very early age developed. Articulation and pronunciation were separated from "language" and were often taught by a speech teacher in a room other than the classroom. There, often before the child had any fluency in spoken language, individual speech sounds might be "worked on," but this work seldom had a positive carryover and there was little integration of the sounds worked on in these speech lessons into any spontaneous spoken language that the child might have. This practice led to children concentrating on "how" to speak rather than on "what" they wanted to say.

In light of today's knowledge of how children with normal hearing learn to be proficient users of their mother tongue, (Wells, 1986), it is little wonder that the practices just outlined served to disrupt the normal language learning mechanism of children with a hearing loss and prevented them from becoming fluent in spoken language. It is understandable that this should have been the case before hearing aids were available. What is disturbing is that, for many hearing-impaired children today, in spite of very changed circumstances, the situation has changed little in relation to the opportunity to become competent users of their residual hearing and, consequently, of spoken language.

It would be wrong to move on to the 1960s without mentioning the work of early pioneers in the field of Parent Guidance. This work developed steadily in the immediate postwar period on both sides of the Atlantic, for example, in the work of the Ewings in Manchester (1954) and that of Pollack (1951) and Beebe (1953) in the United States. Parents were led to realize the value of the use of the residual hearing of their young child with a hearing impairment. This highlighted the need for earlier diagnosis and the early fitting of appropriate hearing aids. Children from these programs were linguistically more capable by school entry age than those whose parents had not been trained in the use of hearing aids and in the ways of maximizing the child's residual hearing. Many parents began to feel that traditional schools for the deaf were inappropriate places for their child who was hearing impaired.

The 1960s

Without doubt the first major advance came with the availability of modern hearing aids. These began to be available in the late 1950s but their general effect was not really felt until the 1960s.

It is difficult to describe all the ways in which the new small body-worn hearing aids changed the educational situation. One effect that was immediately noticeable was the effect on the *educational placement* of children with a hearing loss. Many children with moderate hearing losses, who had previously attended special schools, were able to take their places in their regular neighborhood school with little or no support.

Others, some of whom had severe to profound hearing losses, moved out into classes or special units attached to regular schools in which there was a teacher of the deaf to offer support. Rooms were often fitted with induction loop systems, which helped to overcome the problem of distance from the microphone. Within this setting, there were varying degrees of integration into regular classes. Children so placed had access to the regular curriculum and had much more opportunity to achieve academically than they had previously had. Socially they were in contact with a much wider section of the school population and their behavior was expected to conform to the norm for that population. It was during these years that support services for children in regular schools began to develop.

It was not only within these new settings that the opportunity to use residual hearing existed. Within the Schools for the Deaf the *possibility of using hearing* was actually even greater because, not only were individual hearing aids available, but hard-wired group amplification systems were installed in most classrooms (Ross, 1986). Unfortunately, in many places, these were not used to their full potential nor maintained as well as they should have been. On the whole, teachers understood little about exploiting residual hearing and still relied on the children's eyes as the main way "in" for language. Many considered any benefit the child received from a hearing aid as a bonus, but did not look upon it as an essential.

In the area of *Parent Guidance* the availability of small, modern, body-worn hearing aids brought about big changes. Early intervention began to appear a realistic possibility and more programs developed on both sides of the Atlantic, for example, the work of Whetnall and Fry (1964) in London and, in Denver, that of Pollack (1985) was expanding in its influence at this time. Parents accepted the small hearing aids much more readily than the old cumbersome valve hearing aids. As a result many young children with severe and profound hearing losses developed good listening skills and *began to follow the pattern of language learning of the child with normal hearing, albeit at a later age.* The need to use normal connected language at a normal rate of utterance became obvious, as children with severe and profound hearing losses responded initially to patterns of intonation and began to produce these in the same way as their normally hearing counterparts before any attempts at specific words developed.

Observation of young children with hearing loss all over the world, who have had appropriate hearing aids fitted at an early age, shows that they follow the same pattern of linguistic development as do children with normal hearing. Such evidence makes a mockery of the claim that the natural language of children who are deaf is sign language. The mother tongue of any child is the language of the home and for children who are hearing impaired, born to two normally hearing parents, the mother tongue is spoken language.

The success of children in the early Parent Guidance programs resulted in greater efforts being made to diagnose the hearing loss at an earlier age and *screening programs* were developed for babies around the age of eight to nine months in an attempt to lead to the early identification of those with hearing problems.

The 1960s were years of great expectation. The quality of hearing aids continued to improve and the early results of their use in certain settings gave grounds for real optimism. Toward the end of that decade, the term "deaf" began to be questioned. For centuries that word had had the connotation of "not being able to hear" and had been linked to the concept of "dumb—not being able to speak." Through the use of hearing aids, large numbers of children were demonstrating their ability to hear in varying degrees according to their hearing loss. The term *"hearing impaired"* began to replace *"deaf"* because it was deemed a more positive term and emphasized a child's ability to hear something. In Britain, both schools for the Deaf and schools for the Partially Hearing began to change their names. A common term was used for both, namely, School for the Hearing Impaired.

The 1970s

Throughout the 1970s, the population of the former Schools for the Partially Hearing began to change rapidly. Children with severe and profound hearing losses took the places of the many others who left to go into regular schools. In fact, by the end of that decade, it was impossible in many areas to distinguish, by hearing loss, between the population of the former Schools for the Deaf and those of the former Schools for the Partially Hearing. A practical example of this was the situation in the Birkdale School in England, formerly designated a Partially Hearing School that developed into a school in which only 13% of the population had mean hearing losses under 90 dB. It was therefore considered appropriate that the blanket term "hearing impaired" should cover the whole range of hearing loss. At the same time, it is important to note that *the environments* of what were formerly Schools for the Deaf and those of the former Schools for the Partially Hearing were often still very different.

During the 1970s more and more children began to make full use of their residual hearing, but it was also in this decade that an awareness grew of great discrepancies between the use of hearing to be found in different groups of children. Large numbers of children using their hearing well were coming through to a level of competence in spoken language that was functional for life in society at large. In addition, most of these children were achieving academically as far as their innate ability would allow.

In sharp contrast to this were the groups of children who were not using hearing well although they had the same degree of deafness and the same access to hearing aids and systems of amplification. Educational standards, for the most part, remained low within these groups as could be shown from surveys of reading levels.

Attempts were made to explain away the differences in such groups of children by attributing these to factors inherent in the children themselves. It was claimed that the children in the "non-listening" group had more hearing loss, came from poorer social backgrounds, and were less intelligent, than those who developed good listening skills with resultant competence in spoken language and good levels of attainment. The breakdown of figures for the population of a school like Birkdale School, however, belies this. The children sent to that school were there because it was felt that they would not cope in regular schools with the limited support available at that time. They were certainly no specially selected group.

Their attainments in the English external examination system for High School students shows that this population of "listening, talking" children with a hearing loss were holding their own with their normally hearing counterparts in their academic achievements.

The only area remaining to be investigated was that of the linguistic and educational environments of the two groups, namely, children who were placed in programs where the maximum use was made of their residual hearing (either in Inclusion Programs or in Auditory Special Schools such as Birkdale) and children who remained in more traditional settings where emphasis on looking was predominant. Unfortunately, no one has ever conducted a full scale research into this area, but those who were working in the 1970s, as those in the field today, gradually became aware that the different systems were producing two distinctly different populations of deaf adults (i.e., the "looking deaf" and the "listening deaf"). The listening deaf were developing socially acceptable spoken language and, therefore, when they left school, they had *choice*. They could operate as *independent adults* in society at large or, if they so wished, they could learn sign language to enable them to mix in the Deaf community. The same could not be said for many of the "looking deaf," who were, for the most part, dependent on the services of interpreters when they wished to interact with normally hearing people who did not know sign language. The signing deaf found it too difficult to learn to speak with functionally intelligible speech after leaving school.

Technological advances in the 1970s were significant. During this decade, a good range of reliable and powerful postaural hearing aids became available and gradually replaced the old body-worn aids. At this time, too, FM systems, which cut out the distance between speaker and listener, came into their own. Both of these developments were of particular significance to the ever increasing number of children placed in regular schools as well as those working in Parent Guidance programs.

A greater awareness grew in the 1970s of the need for maintenance services for the audiological equipment, although there was no universal spread of efficient maintenance backup. Even today this varies greatly from area to area.

As hearing aids became more powerful, there was need to develop better quality ear molds and much work was done in that area in this decade.

A new development in the field was the cochlear implant. At this early stage of its development, most of the candidates for implantation were postlingually deafened adults; few children were implanted in these early years.

It is interesting that it was in the 1970s that many developing countries began to show awareness of the needs of their handicapped children. Professionals from developed countries had done work in poorer countries over the years before this but, in the 1970s many approaches were made by developing countries anxious that a better way of life should be available for the children in their midst who were deaf. One outstanding example of this is the program that began in Anadolu University in Eskisehir, Turkey in 1979. From the start, the university made it clear that it wanted the program to lead the children to the ability to speak for themselves, and over the years, it has developed into a vibrant auditory program that achieves good academic results.

By the end of this decade the situation had begun to polarize. Dissatisfied with the results of traditional oralism, some educators, under the influence of the philosophy of Total Communication, officially accepted the practice of adding finger-spelling and/or signing to the old oral approach, claiming that they would continue to encourage the use of hearing aids and speech. Forecasts were made of the way in which standards would rise due to the addition of the manual element.

In complete contrast, other educators, also seeking higher standards, turned their eyes to the work of the psycholinguists who were, at that time, looking more carefully than ever at the language development of normally hearing children. These educators sought to bring about, for hearing-impaired children, conditions that would replicate as nearly as possible the experience of normally hearing children at the language-learning stage. Obviously, this involved even more reliance on the use of residual hearing because the sense of hearing plays such an important part in the normal language-learning process.

The 1980s

During the 1980s, *advances continued in hearing aid technology.* The previously limited use of real-ear measurements developed. There were advances in the knowledge of earmold acoustics, which gave rise to variations in the molds themselves and in the tubing. A wider range of hearing aids than ever before became available, placing a greater weight of responsibility on those prescribing hearing aids to ensure that the most appropriate aids were selected for each child.

The most significant audiological advance at this time, however, was the increasing number of children being put forward for *cochlear implants.* Guidelines were drawn up for the population for whom these were considered appropriate. Multichannel implants began to supplant the single-channel system and the age range for whom the implant was considered was gradually lowered. In addition, it was in this decade children born deaf were included in implant programs. This was a time when the importance of good follow-up in the nature of efficient rehabilitation programs became increasingly obvious.

Parent guidance programs began to be affected by the results of work in normal child language development. An awareness was growing that conversations have a certain structure and that mothers of children with normal hearing seem, unconsciously, to lay the foundations for the development of this, through the way in which they communicate with their child (Bruner, 1983). As a result this caused many seeking to help parents of children with a hearing loss to concentrate their efforts on helping parents *to develop good communication skills rather than to concentrate on teaching specific vocabulary at the early stages.* Making the maximum use of residual hearing was always basic to these programs.

Perhaps the 1980s will be remembered most of all as the time when programs were assessed in an effort to determine if one approach to the education of hearing-impaired children was more effective than another. In the United States, a nationwide study brought to light the fact that the hopes of those who had adopted Total Communication in their programs had not been realized (Geers, Moog, & Schick, 1984). Most children within these programs did not talk *and* sign. Sign took precedence and their skill in that medium was superior to that in spoken language. The children from the oral-only programs had significantly better spoken language production than their peers in the TC programs.

Nor had the addition of the manual element raised academic standards. Paul (1988) makes this clear when he writes,

> Since the 1970s most deaf children have been educated in Total Communication programs . . . Despite improvement in the development of tests, early amplification and the implementation of early intervention or preschool programs, most students are still functionally illiterate upon graduation from high school.

This was not an isolated finding. A study by Quigley and Kretschmer (1982) showed that, without doubt "oral only was best." They found this difficult to accept and sought to explain it away because the oral-only children were seen to have more advantageous backgrounds. Others (McAnally, Rose, & Quigley, 1987) felt that the conditions required to implement auditory/oral programs were too difficult to achieve. They claimed, "oral-aural approaches are difficult to use and seem to require special conditions for success, conditions that cannot easily be met in the public school system."

The Birkdale figures, given earlier, are proof that it is indeed possible to implement an auditory/oral approach with consistently good hearing aid maintenance and management, in an interactive, auditory/oral language environment both at home and at school with a completely unselected group of hearing-impaired children. What is more, many achieve well academically within it.

Throughout the 1980s, there was a continuing trend for more and more hearing-impaired children to enter regular schools. The number of children in special schools decreased rapidly. Toward the end of that decade, concern increased about the effectiveness of some of the inclusion programs. Unless acoustic conditions allowed the children to use their hearing aids effectively and unless staff training was given to those teaching the hearing-impaired children in regular schools, many of these children would not become proficient in spoken language nor in the curriculum. On both sides of the Atlantic, there were laws entitling children who are hearing impaired to support, if their parents opted to have them in the regular school. It was difficult on many occasions to find appropriate and adequate support, but it was significant that the legal requirement was there.

The 1990s

Cochlear implant programs began to cater to a larger number of children and became more diverse. The device itself became smaller. Professionals became more skilled in the rehabilitation work within these programs. The implant began to be offered at a younger age than ever before, thus bringing the child into the world of sound at an earlier age and into language at a time when children with normal hearing are developing theirs.

More and more countries began to develop Early Intervention programs and, within these, parents learned how to manage and maintain the young child's hearing aids/implants and how to interact with their hearing-impaired child in a language-enabling way.

It is little wonder then that dissatisfaction arose with the results of programs that adopted the Total Communication philosophy. In the Canossian School for the hearing impaired in Singapore, a school where it was applied in a truly "total" way, it was found that sign took precedence over speech and that functional spoken language did not develop. The children discarded their hearing aids in situations outside of class and communicated with each other in sign rather than in spoken language.

In situations like this, it became obvious that young people leaving Total Communication programs were not ready for life in society at large. And so, in the 1990s, an even more polarized situation arose than ever before. Poor results, such as those reported from the Total Communication philosophy, resulted in the development of a new approach known as *Bilingualism.* This is a reaction against not only auditory/oral programs, but also against Total Communication, which the Bilingualists see to be speech centered. The proponents of Bilingualism claim that speech does not serve the development of the communication and linguistic needs of the child who is hearing impaired. They hope to offer the sign language of the deaf community as a first language and to introduce verbal language as a second language only after sign language has become well established. There is also the feeling that the emphasis should be on reading and written language rather than on speech.

At a time when possibilities for the use of residual hearing were never greater, it is hard to understand this movement. Today's technology and an increased knowledge regarding optimum conditions for mother tongue learning, can combine to ensure that the auditory option is a realistic one for today's hearing-impaired children. It is our professional responsibility to ensure that in every area, this auditory option is available.

The 21st Century

As we enter a new century, the introduction of neonatal screening is helping to identify deafness at a much earlier age than ever before and preparations are being made to train professionals for work with the parents of very young children who are identified as having a hearing loss. This should have repercussions on the opportunities afforded to babies born with a hearing loss to develop spoken language, because they should be fitted with hearing aids at an age when a child with normal hearing is learning language, so they will not spend long in a silent world.

New programmable and digital hearing aids are offering superior listening conditions to many children and this, in turn, has a marked effect on the quality of their spoken language. The success of cochlear implant programs is providing those for whom conventional hearing aids do not supply enough information the opportunity to hear and learn language in the same way as a normally hearing child. Never has the chance for children with a hearing loss to develop fluent spoken language been so great.

In spite of this, many people today are trying to ensure that everything is "politically correct" and are guarding the rights of minority groups. The traditional adult deaf are exerting pressure on decision makers in the field of education. Their plea is for the retention of sign language programs on the grounds that, without them, the so-called Deaf community will disappear (Lane & Bahan, 1998).

At the same time, however, there is a growing awareness of the need for a worldwide movement to support the ever increasing number of young people, who, in spite of severe and profound hearing losses, are using their residual hearing to its full potential and are reaching levels of spoken language that enable them to mix freely in wider society and make friends within it. In such a group we find young people who are achieving well academically and are gaining entrance to normal universities if they have that kind of innate ability. There is no doubt that they have special needs, for example, the services of oral interpreters or note takers, but they have developed the linguistic ability to live independent lives. For those who would not have gone to university had they not been deaf, there are many more job opportunities than for their counterparts from signing programs who cannot function independently linguistically. It is important that the rights of these listening, talking young people are defended.

APPENDIX B

Parent Guidance Report Form

Name: _____   Date: _____

1. Checking of hearing instruments (including FM)

   _____

   _____

   _____

2. Caregiver interaction

   a. Material used: _____

      _____

   b. Comments: _____

      _____

      _____

      _____

      _____

3. Therapist interaction

   a. Material used: _____

      _____

   b. Comments: _____

      _____

      _____

      _____

      _____

4. Child's communicative behavior

   a. General: _____

      _____

      _____

      _____

   b. Auditory responses: _____

      _____

      _____

      _____

c. Receptive language: _____

_____

_____

_____

d. Expressive language—nonverbal: _____

_____

_____

_____

e. Expressive language—verbal: _____

_____

_____

_____

5. Advice/suggestions offered:

_____

_____

_____

6. Plan for next visit:

_____

_____

_____

Index

143